MIRIAM VERHEYDEN

Everything Is Broken and Completely Fine

Mental Illness, Quitting Alcohol, and Living through Unprecedented Times

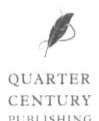

QUARTER
CENTURY
PUBLISHING

First published by Quarter Century Publishing 2023

Copyright © 2023 by Miriam Verheyden

All rights reserved. No part of this publication may be reproduced, stored or transmitted in any form or by any means, electronic, mechanical, photocopying, recording, scanning, or otherwise without written permission from the publisher. It is illegal to copy this book, post it to a website, or distribute it by any other means without permission.

Miriam Verheyden asserts the moral right to be identified as the author of this work.

Miriam Verheyden has no responsibility for the persistence or accuracy of URLs for external or third-party Internet Websites referred to in this publication and does not guarantee that any content on such Websites is, or will remain, accurate or appropriate.

First edition

This book was professionally typeset on Reedsy.
Find out more at reedsy.com

For Lily

Contents

Foreword	iii
Preface	iv
Prologue	1
The Happily Ever After	6
Is He Losing His Mind, Or Am I?	12
Lyme Disease	20
Depression	28
Depression and Alcohol	34
Going Away	41
Sober Curious	51
PMDD	62
Don't Should All Over Yourself	70
COVID-19	80
Cheers to the World Ending	88
Gifts	96
Therapy I	100
Puppies	109
Great Expectations	115
Surrounded by Fire	124
Protests	131
Therapy II	137
Flood	146
And Just Like That	155
Grey Area Drinking	165
The Goopy Stage	174
Keynote Speaker	184

Lily	194
Surviving and Thriving with Mental Illness	205
Epilogue	213
Acknowledgments	215
About the Author	216
Also by Miriam Verheyden	217

Foreword

This is a true story. I have changed the names and identifying characteristics of everyone to protect their identities. The only real names are the ones of my husband Richard and my dogs.

Events described in the hospitals have been altered for privacy reasons. I've also slightly condensed the timeline for clarity and better flow of the story.

Preface

What happens *after* the happily ever after? After you got the man, the house, the job, and everything you thought you ever wanted? Movies and fairy tales conveniently end right there, with a last shot of the deliriously happy couple before panning out. Credits, sweeping music, the end.

It's understandable. Who wants to see Cinderella yell at her prince for leaving wet towels on the floor again? Or watch Pretty Woman Vivian get divorced from Edward because he's insufferably controlling?

Even though we know on a rational level that happy endings aren't real, we still believe that the key to happiness is getting everything we want. After all, that's what we're being promised by clever advertisements and the gentle brainwashing of modern media: become successful, rich, thin, find the perfect partner, live in the perfect house, and you will be happy forever.

Spoiler: it's a lie.

I've been obsessed with happiness all my life. It was my standard answer to the question "what do you want to be when you grow up?", and my main criteria as a teenager when it came to career plans: "I just want to do something that makes me happy." I cared little about money, prospects, or suitability, believing that happiness trumped them all. The reason for my preoccupation with happiness is that I've been carrying around a dark secret for most of my life. I was an anxious child who constantly worried: about my parents dying, about turning blind, about a third world war, about people not liking me. I also experienced periods of profound sadness, and a world weariness so heavy that it was almost impossible for me to get out of bed sometimes. For many years I had no idea what was wrong with me. I was led to believe that I was an ungrateful overthinker who took herself way too seriously and spent indecent amounts of time worrying about herself. My parents didn't believe in anxiety and depression, at least not for their daughter who had "no reason to be depressed", and they'd prescribe more work so "you don't have time to think so much". I grew up believing something was wrong with my personality, and I resolved to hide the dark side of me and hope nobody else would ever find it.

At 23 I moved to Canada, the land of my dreams, to be with the man of my dreams. Still a firm believer in the happily ever after, I put high hopes into this move, expecting that I'd left my demons behind in Germany, never to be bothered by them again.

That didn't happen.

Over the next ten years as I learnt a new language, settled into my role as wife and stepmother, went back to school and found my footing in a new country, I was still plagued by strange episodes I couldn't control. At times I would be hit by a rage so intense, I was screaming unspeakable things at my husband, convinced he was the worst man in the world. At other times I'd lie listlessly on the couch, unable to focus on a book or TV, staring at the ceiling and wondering what the point was of everything. Life seemed to be an endless slog of boring, exhausting days with no colour or joy. I felt like I was stuck in a waiting room, where the wait was excruciating but being called would mean The End, and I didn't know what was worse – the waiting or for everything to be over?

Luckily, my "moods" would always fade after a while. We barely spoke about them, and I was halfway convinced that I was hiding them pretty well. We all had bad days, right? When I wasn't in one of my "moods" I was cheerful, bubbly, happy and full of life. Everything was *fine*.

But when I cried every day on a vacation in Hawaii and couldn't muster any enthusiasm for the beauty around me, my husband Richard persuaded me that I needed help. Not knowing how to get in touch with a shrink (and not knowing the difference between psychiatrists, psychologists, and therapists) we went to our family doctor. A kind man resembling Santa Claus, he listened patiently to my teary tale, diagnosed depression, and then he offered three astonishing facts: he said that my depression was a) not my fault, b) very common (say what?), and c) treatable.

He explained that the most likely cause of my depression was a chemical imbalance in my brain: a shortage of serotonin, a neurotransmitter. He compared my condition to someone having diabetes, and he said: "You wouldn't feel guilty for having diabetes, would you? Or think that it's your fault? It's the same with depression."

He prescribed me the antidepressant Citalopram, gave me a fatherly pat on the head, and I felt like the weight of the world had been lifted off my shoulders.

The effect of the drug was almost immediate. It felt like a soft blanket settled over me and made everything less harsh. The stormy sea of my emotions was transformed into a calm ocean. I felt a peace that I hadn't felt before. It was amazing!

He hadn't mentioned therapy, so I didn't either. If it was just a chemical imbalance in my brain the pills were all I needed, right? Get some extra serotonin and all is well. I was pretty sure that as long as I took my antidepressants, I was cured. Had I finally arrived at the happy ending I'd been yearning for all my life?

It wasn't to be. The pills alone were about as effective as slapping some duct tape on a broken car and saying it's fixed. I was doing okay for a while, but eventually different car parts were starting to fall off. The duct tape alone couldn't handle the job any longer.

The rage attacks had lessened but never stopped, and when a friend told me about PMDD (Premenstrual Dysphoric Disorder), a condition I had never heard of before, another piece of the puzzle clicked into place.

(You will learn more about PMDD in chapter 9.)

One of the most significant symptoms of PMDD is severe irritability, and there are ways to lessen it. But first you have to know what you are dealing with, and I didn't get this diagnosis until I was 38 years old, five years after my diagnosis of depression.

During the visits with my doctor I never got around to telling him about the intrusive thoughts and irrational fears I was having. I didn't tell him how I couldn't help but regularly envision my husband being dead; how I never stopped worrying about money; how I couldn't stop wondering if everybody hated me; how I either agonized over the past or fretted about the future. I thought I was simply a worrier, not wanting to admit that another mental health condition may be the cause of it. Me, anxious? No way.

It wasn't until 2020 that I finally admitted defeat and sought more help. The antidepressants weren't cutting it anymore in a world that had turned upside down, and I now had another secret that was starting to get too heavy to carry: I was drinking too much.

Living in denial is exhausting. If you believe, wittingly or unwittingly, that a part of you is so deeply flawed that you are unlovable, you will do anything to hide it from others and avoid thinking about it. For someone whose mental illness manifests as intrusive thoughts and a never-ending barrage of insults telling her that she's worthless, this is tricky. What will make the voices stop?

Enter wine. Endorsed by society as the ultimate relaxant, wine seemingly does just that: it blurs the edges, takes away the sharpness of the world and makes everything soft and fuzzy. Most important to me, it managed to shut up the voices in my head telling me how useless I was. For a while I thought wine was the key to transform from a chronic worrier with low self-esteem into a carefree, confident, happy-go- lucky person. I almost felt normal.

But it came at a heavy price.

Alcohol, a known depressant, made my mental health significantly worse. After the short-lived happy feeling my mood would nose-dive sharply. It increased my anxiety and gave me terrible hanxiety (= anxiety caused by a hangover) that caused severe self-loathing. Drinking kept me in depressive episodes longer and would ignite the dreaded PMDD rage like a lit match held too close to kerosene. Instead of solving my low mood, it contributed to it.

This is the story of what happens when you pretend your mental illness doesn't exist – and how your life changes once you accept it. You may recognize yourself in these pages because we all have secrets we don't want anyone else to see. But once we learn to embrace the scariest, darkest parts of ourselves we can release the shame and fear that have weighed so heavily on us.

Did I ever find my happily ever after?

I've found something better. I finally got over that impossible expectation that will always leave you disappointed.

Once you get past it you can ask the important question: what happens *after* the happily ever after?

Everything. You've learnt that every life is a continuation of ups and downs, of good experiences and not so great ones. You have seen, to your utter astonishment, that life can take turns wilder than what you could have ever imagined. You have witnessed people packing several lives into one: selling their house to go back to school in their 30s; starting a new career in their 40s,;quitting their addiction and helping other people in their 50s; moving across the world to work for a non-profit in their 60s; building their first house in their 70s; having a great romance in their 80s.

Life is so much more interesting and so much more unexpected if we let go of our conditioned expectations of what we think we *should* want.

After I finished writing my first book *Let's Pretend This is Normal* in 2017 I thought I'd never write another memoir. I wouldn't have to since I believed to have found my happy ending and nothing noteworthy was going to happen except for bliss and euphoria – great to live in, not interesting enough to write about. But as you will see in the following pages, the story didn't end there.

As I'm sitting here in December of 2022, we are on the brink of our next big adventure: another move to a piece of land that's everything we've ever wanted. It's not anything I could have ever foreseen back in 2017, when I thought I had my future mapped out for the rest of my life. Chapter 2 picks the story up where I left off, and looking back, I'm so grateful things didn't turn out the way I expected them to – because the reality is so much better than I ever thought possible. While this books recounts my life from 2017-2022, the focus is on my mental illness. I wrote it for everyone who also suffers from a mental illness, but maybe even more importantly, I wrote it for their family members and friends. I know how difficult it can be to share your life with someone whose mental health is compromised, not least because we will do our best to hide the extent of it from you. We might appear normal to you most of the time, but then act in what appears to be unpredictable or out of character, which isn't easy to live with.

We do this because there is still a lot of stigma and shame associated with having a mental illness. While our society is making strides to remove the stigma, I can tell you from experience that I'm more forgiving towards someone else having it than towards myself. It's fine for *others* to have anxiety, depression and PMDD, but for me? *I'm* stronger than that.

Well, joke's on me. Turns out, there is no greater strength than facing your challenges and living *with* them instead of against them. For anyone out there who also has a mental illness and continues to get out of bed every day (or most days, let's be real): **you are stronger than you know.**

For everyone who lives with us and loves us, demons and all: we see you, we appreciate you, and we love you more than we'll ever be able to express.

Prologue

The stomach cramps start Friday night. I've taken two Naproxen earlier for the headache I normally never get, and I'm wondering if that's what's giving me the cramps. I feel lousy, so I'm hoping that I won't get called back to the hospital tonight. I'm on call every other weekend, and normally I don't mind getting called in. But tonight I'm in agony, and the thought of having to drag my sorry ass to the hospital and help another person while I'm in so much pain makes me feel even sicker. I go to bed at eight, wishing for sleep to obliterate the pain.

No such luck. I toss and turn restlessly, frequently torn from sleep when a particularly intense cramp is twisting my insides. Two hours after I went to bed I'm woken up by nausea and stumble to the bathroom to throw up. Afterwards I stand at the sink to wash my hands and rinse my mouth, and I'm appalled at my reflection: I'm pale with a green tinge to my skin, my eyes are bloodshot, and I have red spots on my cheeks. My stringy hair is pasted to the side of my head and my hands are shaking. I can't bear to look at myself any longer, so I turn off the light and shuffle back to bed.

I repeat this sad process several more times throughout this endless night, minus looking at myself in the mirror. Fortunately I don't get called in. While I'm staying in bed, carefully massaging my tummy and existing on ginger tea and dry toast, I wonder what could have caused this illness. I don't have the typical diarrhea or fever that comes with a stomach flu. I know that it's not food poisoning, because I had that before, and this is different. Besides, I haven't eaten anything that may cause food poisoning, I'm sure of it. What's going on?

I'm usually a healthy person. I have a robust stomach, no chronic pain to speak of, and my energy levels are decent for a 42-year-old woman with mental illness. But lately I've been off. I had two headaches in a week, which is more than what I ordinarily get in a year. My joints are aching, and I have a constant back ache. I'm exhausted all the time, and I feel weepy and close to tears most days. I've been crying in the car to and from work for no discernible reason. Sometimes it's the burnt trees from last year's wildfires that set me off, sometimes it's when I pass the section on the highway where my car hit ice a couple of months ago and I thought for one terrifying, heart-stopping moment I would slide off the mountain. Sometimes I simply cry because it releases some of the terrible tension inside me.

As soon as I enter my workplace I put the mask on. The mask of being friendly and smiley and cheerful. I've been taught to leave my personal problems at home, to be professional and competent. My mom took it as far as to advise me to "never let them see the real you", which is a philosophy I don't agree with. But being professional at work is sound advice that has served me well. It's been particularly useful working in healthcare over the last two years since the beginning of the pandemic. I've had to listen to rants about the vaccine mandate, conspiracy theories about "the plandemic (pLandemic because it's been planned – get it?) being planted by the UN to eliminate 90% of the world population", complaints about the cancellation of surgeries and reduction of services. People have regaled me at great length with their opinion about how masks are useless and don't do anything, that the vaccine kills or leaves women infertile, how the government is a tyrant and tries to manipulate us all. And all the while I stay polite and noncommittal, provide the service I'm here for and don't yell at them to shut up, which is what I would like to do.

At first I did understand their fears and frustrations. I was sympathetic and patient and I listened, making them feel heard and validated.

But lately it's become more and more difficult. My well of patience has dried up, and I'm genuinely afraid that I will explode on someone. I've been working non-stop through the pandemic. I've driven through burning forests in the summer of 2021. We were evacuated for a week due to the wildfires, worried that we might lose everything. Roads have been closed on me while I was at work, making me panic that I might be cut off from home for days or weeks. We've worked short-staffed for months. I was unofficially put in charge at one of my hospitals with all of the responsibility and none of the compensation.

I was on the highway that got completely destroyed by the flood on the day it happened, the angry water lapping at my tires, pieces of the road already broken off. Could I have fallen in the river and being swept away? I refuse to think about it.

Most people know little about the work of an x-ray technologist. "Don't you just push a button?" Not quite.

I was the one who took the chest x-ray that diagnosed a patient with stage 4 lung cancer. She kept coming back to the ER with complications, and every time I saw her she had lost more weight and looked frailer. Three months later she was dead. I locked myself in the bathroom and cried when I found out.

Right around the same time I x-rayed another patient who had a tumour in his lung. He had waited to come to the hospital because he was afraid of COVID. He also had end- stage lung cancer and passed away a few months later.

One of the nurses I work with is an ICU nurse. Her stories of what it's like to die of COVID are horrific. It's an especially stark contrast when you go from having her stories fresh in your mind to a patient who insists that COVID is fake. I'd love to send these people to her to give them a much-needed dose of reality, but of course I can't. Besides, they probably wouldn't believe her anyway.

And all the while I'm asked to work more.

"Can you help out?"

"You are the only one who is available, can you do it?"

"Please help, please be a friend and team-player."

I keep saying yes, thinking I can do it. I'm strong, I'm resilient, I'm tough. I'm German, I was born and raised to push through, I've worked through period cramps and fevers, through heartbreak and a depression I didn't know

I had. If the world is tough you've gotta be tougher, right?

But every few months my body goes on strike. I will wake up with my neck seized up so painfully that I can't move. I will be bed-bound for a few days, eating muscle relaxers like candy and being secretly grateful for the break.

In 2021 I got such a severe, sharp pain in my upper left back that I was afraid I was having a heart attack. I went to the ER and got thoroughly checked out by my favourite doctor who wanted to make sure he didn't miss anything. There was nothing wrong with me physically. I stayed for several hours until the pain had faded and was sent home with strict instructions to come right back should it start again.

I was back at work the next day.

In 2020 I lost my voice for four days. It was completely gone. My husband had to call in sick for me because I was mute.

In December of that year a friend committed suicide and my mother-in-law died four days later. I didn't miss a single day of work.

In 2019 I woke up during another on-call weekend feeling like death warmed over: my entire body ached, I had stomach pains, I was hot and cold and shivery. I went to the emergency department of that hospital, got checked over, and again they couldn't find anything. The doctor gave me a shot of Toradol and told me to rest, promising that she would try not to call me in. I went home and slept the entire weekend.

Now it's 2022, and I'm having these mystery stomach cramps that won't go away. I call in sick for my shift on Monday and the pain eases a little.

On Tuesday I have therapy and boy do I need it. I start crying before I can even say hello, and she listens with great compassion. I love my therapist, and right now she's what's keeping me going. She's my life raft in the storm, and I cling on with all my might. I'm telling her much of what I've recounted just now, and also the shameful secret I've been keeping: I've been contemplating to take a leave from work. It feels like the ultimate failure, and my parents would be appalled.

But I'm depleted. I have nothing left in me to give. I'm mentally depleted and physically sick. My therapist encourages me to take the break I need. And then she says this: "You've been limping along with one leg in a bear trap.

You have to stop. You're bleeding out. You can't go on like this anymore."

As soon as we are done I call my family doctor for an emergency appointment. Later that day, with much sobbing (I can't seem to stop crying) I tell him about my physical symptoms and the disaster zone that's my mental health. He diagnoses burnout and recommends taking a month off work. The next day I call work and arrange for the time off. I'm riddled with guilt and a profound sense of failure – lots to talk about in my next therapy session.

It's done. And I suddenly notice that my stomach pain that started six days ago is gone.

I swear my body is breathing a sigh of relief. *It's about time you listened to me*, I imagine it saying. *I didn't know how to make it any clearer.*

Seeing it all written out like this, the signposts spelling out that I was doing too much have been there all along. But I didn't see them. I thought all the good advice about self-care and putting the oxygen mask on first were for other, weaker people. I assumed I was tougher than them. I liked to say that I had a mental illness, it didn't have me. My self-worth was so tightly bound to being hard-working and not lazy, the thought of having to take time off work was terrifying.

Until I didn't have a choice. Turns out that my body is stronger than my will. Smarter, too, which is a good thing. My brain can't always be trusted because it's not healthy. You wouldn't run a race with a broken leg, would you? I've been relying on a broken brain to make sound choices for me.

No more. I've stepped off the treadmill. I'm still. And I'm taking a goddamn break.

The Happily Ever After

We are sitting by the huge windows in our new house, surrounded by cardboard boxes, sipping coffee, and watching the sunrise. We have a front-row seat to the sunrise from these windows which is amazing! After a while, Richard touches my arm and points to something outside. A group of deer is moving gracefully over our property, stopping here and there for a nibble of dry grass. We both keep watching quietly, holding hands.

"Is this really our life now?" I whisper.

"It sure is," he replies and squeezes my hand. As I'm gazing outside, I suddenly get a powerful sense of déjà vu. I feel certain that I've experienced this exact moment before. But I also know for a fact that I've never woken up in this house before, and Richard and I haven't been anywhere like this. I ponder for a while why this feels so familiar, and then it comes to me.

The picture.

Two years ago, I wrote a blog post called *Chasing liquid gold*.

It's about a hunting trip Richard went on with a buddy where he experiences floating ice crystals in the air. When they're lit up by the sun it looks like liquid gold is suspended in the air, and according to Richard it's a magical experience. I don't experience FOMO often, but when I heard him gushing about it (and he is not a man who gushes) I was quite jealous. I would have *loved* to see that. But FOMO aside, it sparked our desire to move again.

We've been playing with the idea of moving to somewhere wilder for years. Our neighbourhood is nice, but it looks like suburbia with slightly larger yards. It's all very tidy and urbane and tame. We are craving more wilderness, less picture-perfect lawns. In fact, not having a lawn is on the top of our wish list – we are both sick to death of mowing the lawn.

I had attached a picture to that post. It was a drawing of a winter scene at night, with a half-moon in the sky. You are looking at a gently downhill sloping yard with scattered pine trees, all covered in a thick layer of fluffy, picturesque snow. There's a fence with an owl perched on top of it, and a black dog stands on the path leading away from the yard, looking towards an approaching light that's coming from around a hedge. In the distance are snow-covered mountains shimmering silver in the moonlight.

Our view is reminding me of that picture. I pull up the post on my phone to show Richard, and I'm astonished by the similarities. The drawing looks like it was inspired by the very view I'm looking at right now. Then I notice something else: I wrote it *exactly* two years ago. To the day. I start reading, and I'm getting goosebumps: we've got a *lot* of the things I described in that post, even though I hadn't thought of it throughout our house hunting process.

Wow.

I lean back, momentarily speechless. Do dreams come true or *what*?

It just keeps getting better. In February I'm hired at the local hospital. After an adjustment period where I feel a bit lonely and miss my old work family, I fall in love with the concept of a rural hospital. Everything is so much more chill than it was in any of the other hospitals I worked before. For starters, everybody calls the doctors by their first name. Can you believe that? After a few months and lots of internal debate, I try it out one day, half expecting to be reprimanded and told to call them **Doctor** So-and-so. To my delight it doesn't happen. For the first time in my life, I chat with doctors just like I do with other people, without getting nervous or stammering or saying something stupid. It's a revelation to get to know these guys better and to realize that they are just ordinary people. Who knew? I grew up seeing my parents act deferentially towards anyone who they believed was "above" them: doctors, lawyers, academics. Even though I believe that we are all equals, I had internalized those lessons more than I wanted to. It's not until now that I'm actively unlearning this behaviour.

In May our social life explodes. Before our move I had expected to see less people than before since we now lived in the "wilderness". I was in equal measures excited and apprehensive about living a life of more solitude and introspection. In my daydreams I saw myself as a real writer who would spend days on end with only her husband and dogs as company, writing and contemplating the mysteries of the universe and her strange, complicated mind.

The reality looks laughably different; our everyday life is positively lousy with people.

There are the neighbours we see daily and hang out with at least once a week; the carpenter who has been working five days a week at our place for the last month and a half; a standing weekly dinner date with a group of guys in our old town (we attend at least twice a month); and a stream of overnight visitors from our old life that at first trickled in but is now turning into a flood of guests.

Then there are the cowboys that Richard attracts like honey attracts flies, guys who pull up in beat-up pickup trucks, wearing plaid shirts and cowboy hats, asking me politely to see "my old man" to look at animals and talk about cattle prices.

Sooner or later they usually end up sitting in the sunshine with cold cans of beer in hand, telling jokes while country music is playing. None of these guys travels without a well- stocked cooler full of beer, and their supply of jokes is just as well stocked.

"Did you know that Willie Nelson died?"

We are all shocked. "What, really?"

"Yes, he was playing *On the Road Again*."

A moment's collective silence until realization dawns, and then we burst out laughing.

(At the time of me writing this, Willie Nelson is alive and well.)

Sooner or later come the toasts:

"Here's to the women in the high-heeled shoes,
  they spend my money and drink my booze,

they lost their cherry but that's no sin,
because they still have the box the cherry came in."

"Here's to the women we love best,
many a times I sucked their chest.
I fucked them smiling, I fucked them crying,
if they had wings, I'd fuck them flying."

My first reaction to the last toast is *what the fuck* – quickly followed by what I've conditioned myself to be: easy-going with a sense of humour. Jokes about having sex with crying women – hahaha, how hilarious! It's all in good fun, right? No need to spoil a good time by getting annoyingly feminist, that would be such a downer. The guys would all look at my poor husband with pity, feeling sorry for him for having such a humourless wife. Besides, the joke-teller apologized in advance the first time he was telling a dirty joke and asked if I'm okay with it, and I assured him that I am. Fun and easy-going, remember? You know what else helps with the discomfort? Alcohol. After a few beers everything seems funny. The guys tell Richard how lucky he is for having such a beautiful and cool wife, and I love them. Who cares if they are making misogynistic jokes? They are from a different generation; they don't even know that this is bad. It's F-U-N-N-Y Miriam, not insulting to women. Don't take everything so serious all the time.

Besides, it's all such a throwback to the times as a kid when I watched old Westerns with my dad, I can't help but love everything: the cheap beer, the weathered cowboys, the country music, and the fact that we are sitting on hay bales because we don't have enough chairs.

There's a warm atmosphere of camaraderie and belonging, and for someone who has never felt like she truly belonged anywhere this is the best gift in the world.

As summer progresses so does the feeling of being on permanent vacation. I work part-time, write most days, and still have enough time to hang out with our new friends. I've never felt happier or more carefree.

On hot days you can find us sitting in the shade, enjoying the warm breeze and a cold drink, resting until it gets cooler. Animals and humans alike come alive again in the early evening, when Richard and I are doing chores and watch the dogs and horses play exuberantly, creating billows of dust in their wake.

We walk around half naked, wearing denim cut-offs and Birkenstock sandals and are soon sporting matching striped tans on our feet.

My hair is windblown, my face full of freckles and my eyes are sparkling. I fall asleep with a smile on my face and wake up excited for the day, having breakfast with hummingbirds every morning.

I keep the windows and front door open all day for three months straight to have the warm breeze blow its delicious smell of sun-drenched pine and desert into the house. The dogs run in and out like little kids, and the occasional chicken wanders in as well, squawking indignantly when I chase it back outside.

A fine layer of dust covers everything in the house, but I don't care. I like having a piece of the desert in my house, just like a proper beach house should contain a good amount of sand on its floors. Besides, our new house is small enough that I can clean the whole thing in an hour.

In July I fly to Paris for a quick city trip with my sister.

I finish the first draft of my book *Let's Pretend This is Normal.* In August we float down the river on inner tubes, with an extra inner tube rigged with netting to hold our booze. One of the guys is chosen as the bartender and holds on to the "bar" by a string the entire time, throwing us fresh cans when ours are empty.

Richard and I tell each other at least once a day how lucky we are.

***

And then September comes.

Richard has booked a trip to Germany for almost three weeks, which is longer than usual because he's not only visiting his mom but also going on a week-long vacation to Mallorca with his buddies.

The weekend before he leaves we have our yearly rodeo in town, and we decide to go.

I get dressed up for the event: I curl my hair and put on a little white lace dress and my favourite cowboy booties. Richard is wearing a light-blue plaid shirt that brings out the blue of his eyes, form-fitting jeans, cowboy boots, and his white summer hat. We both look tan and happy, and we enjoy the rodeo tremendously.

As we are heading back to our truck, I am struck by the beauty of our surroundings: the golden hue of the sun-bleached grass in the meadow in front of us, with the green trees behind and the blue sky above creating the perfect backdrop.

"Let's take a quick photo," I say, pulling Richard along.

I put my camera on the back of someone's truck parked by the meadow and direct Richard to the best spot. Then I set the timer to ten seconds burst mode and hurry to Richard's side. It's my favourite way to snap photos of us without relying on anybody else.

We do only one set.

It's *perfect*. I end up using one of the photos as cover for my first book.

It's the last perfect moment of the summer.

Is He Losing His Mind, Or Am I?

"Hey, whatshisname just called," he says, and then falls silent.

"Who?" I ask impatiently. "And what did they want? Use your words." I'm scared, and when I get scared, I get short-tempered. It's an unfortunate character flaw I need to work on.

Richard has been losing his words. Some of his sentences are incomprehensible, like this one for example: "Whatshisname called and talked to me about..." [pause] [pause continues] [pause gets uncomfortably long] "damn it, I forgot."

It's worrying. He's 63 years old. His dad had dementia. My grandma had Alzheimer's. We've both witnessed the awful mental decline of loved ones and it was horrible to watch. The fear in their eyes when they didn't know where they were. The confusion when they had no idea who these people were that claimed to be their wife or husband. My father-in-law, who always recognized his son's voice on the phone, called us once and told Richard: "There's a woman sitting on the table across from me, and I don't know who she is. I think she's keeping me prisoner. And you won't believe it – she's wearing your mother's wedding ring. Who is she? Why is she doing this? I want to leave. I want to go home."

He was born in his house and had never lived anywhere else. He had been married to my mother-in-law for over 50 years. He wanted to go to a place that only existed in his mind – the home of his childhood. It was heartbreaking.

And now here is Richard, my beloved husband, who can't find words for the simplest things. Names are all but lost to him. When I call him at lunchtime and ask if he ate breakfast, he can't remember. When he picks up the phone to call a friend, he forgets who it is he's calling or what he wanted to talk about by the time they pick up. More than once I've seen him struggle through a conversation, sometimes not knowing who it is he's talking to.

"I didn't want to ask who it is because I was the one calling him," he confides after one of those conversations. "It wasn't until he mentioned his wife Emma that I knew who it was."

"Next time tell me who you are going to call so I can help you," I instruct him, and that's what we do. I become his second, more dependable brain since we can't rely on his own right now.

We don't say it out loud, but we are both thinking the same: is Richard in the early stages of Alzheimer's disease?

I'm extremely stressed out about it. In the evening I open a bottle of wine, plunk myself down in front of the computer and google "early signs of dementia". The results are not good: memory loss, difficulty communicating or finding words, difficulty problem-solving, difficulty with planning or organizing, confusion. Fuck! They all apply. I take a big gulp and continue reading, my dread growing: personality changes, depression, anxiety, agitation.

My own anxiety and agitation rise with every word that I read, and tears are filling my eyes. I'm thirty-seven years old and my husband may have dementia. I can't deal with this. What am I going to do? Will I have to give up my job and become his caregiver? What will we do for money? Will he have to go to a care facility at some stage? WHAT AM I GOING TO DO?

I reach for the wine bottle to top up my glass and see that it's empty. Oopsy daisy, how did that happen?

Never mind. I go to the living room where Richard's lying on the couch, watching TV.

"How are you feeling?" I ask him softly and squeeze myself onto the couch next to him.

"My knee is still really bugging me," he says.

"Oh?" I'm not concerned about his knee; I'm worried about his mind.

Richard has been limping ever since he came back from Germany, but he's had aches and pains for as long as I've known him. Something's always hurting him, but I've chalked it up to him being a man suffering from a wide variety of man colds.

"Yeah, it must be from the pork and beer I had in Germany. Maybe it's my arthritis acting up."

"Do you want me to make an appointment with the doctor?"

"Yes, you better."

"Okay, I'll call him first thing tomorrow," I promise, give him a kiss, and go to bed.

A week later we are sitting in our doctor's office. I came with Richard because of the unreliability of his memory, and his general ineptitude in medical surroundings. His typical answer to the doctor's question "how are you feeling?" is "fine", which is not quite detailed enough.

Together we explain his knee pain and his history of joint pain. Richard thinks his body has a sensitivity to pork, so he usually doesn't eat it; but he's powerless against the temptation of currywurst, pork sausage with a spicy tomato-curry sauce that he eats several times every time he's in Germany.

"I think it's just my arthritis acting up, but this time it's worse than usual," he tells the doctor.

"Have you changed anything else about your diet?" he asks, and Richard mentions the beer he drank while on vacation.

"I usually don't drink beer because it doesn't sit well with me. But I had a few with my buddies while I was there."

The doctor nods understandingly. "I'm going to order x-rays of your knees and prescribe you a round of Indomethacin. It's probably gout, and the medication should take care of that."

Neither of us mentions his memory problems. If we don't talk about it, we can pretend that it doesn't exist. Maybe it isn't that bad and we're just overreacting? Let's focus on the problem that can be fixed with pills first.

Except that the pills don't help at all. After the five days of medication are over the pain is still there, worse than before. It's also developed a new trick: it's moving around his body now. From his right knee to his left, and it sometimes hangs out in his right elbow for a while just for kicks. When that happens, he can't lift his teacup with his right hand, let alone anything heavier. It makes doing chores difficult.

I ask him to describe the pain to me. "Is it sharp, dull, hot, stabbing?"

Richard shrugs his shoulders helplessly. "I can't describe it, but it's awful. Worse than anything I've ever had before."

I make another appointment with our doctor.

"It's not gout," he summarizes succinctly. "His knee x-rays look good," he continues, "but let's order some more joint x-rays. I'll also refer you to a rheumatologist. It sounds like arthritis to me, and a rheumatologist will be able to treat it."

"I had juvenile arthritis as a kid," Richard says unexpectedly. What? Did I know that? I don't think so.

"Why didn't you say so before?" I ask accusingly. I feel like we failed a test or something in front of the doctor. I hate that feeling.

"I just remembered. I was in the hospital for a month when I was eight, with the same pain I'm having now. It was terrible."

"So, they diagnosed you with juvenile arthritis?" the doctor asks.

"They didn't really know what it was," Richard replies. "After a month they sent me home. I was in so much pain that my dad had to carry me up the stairs to my room; I couldn't walk. They said the most likely explanation for my pain was juvenile arthritis. I was in bed for a while before it got slowly better over the next few months. I missed so much school that I had to repeat the year."

"How has it been over the years?"

"I was back to playing soccer the year after," Richard reports proudly. "I've had some pain over the years, especially during the winter when we were living at the coast, but nothing like this."

"Okay. I'm going to order some blood tests and the x-rays, and get you fast-tracked to see a rheumatologist."

He also prescribes more anti-inflammatory medication and pills for the pain, and then we are dismissed.

We do everything the doctor tells us to do: Richard gets a ton of blood drawn, inadvertently giving the old bloodletting a go – it's as useless for him as it was in medieval times and doesn't reveal anything bad. According to his blood, Richard is in excellent health. Same goes for his x-rays: his bones and joints are in peak condition for a man his age.

This would all be great news were it not for the fact that he's getting worse every day.

His short-term memory is further deteriorating. We've started watching *Mad Men* every night in an attempt to distract ourselves, and Richard can't keep up with the plot.

He keeps forgetting the characters' names and can't follow the story line. You know it's bad when a man forgets Joan Harris, one of the sexiest women on TV of all time.

He has no appetite and is losing weight at an alarming rate. All he wants to eat is canned peaches, so that's what I buy: canned peaches by the dozen.

He's constantly cold, so we turn up the heat as high as it goes. It's tropical in our home, yet Richard is shivering. Except at night, when he sweats through his clothes and his sheets are literally dripping. We start putting towels on his bed to soak up some of the sweat and avoid having to change the sheets in the middle of the night.

But the worst is the pain. He can't sit for longer than ten minutes before his butt gets numb. When he needs to get up and first puts his feet gingerly on the floor, an intense pain shoots from his ankles up his legs. He often calls for help, and when I pull him up as carefully as I can, he screams in pain. The pain has now spread from his legs and elbow into his shoulders, which means he can't drive a car anymore – it hurts too much to steer.

The only thing that slightly relieves his pain are Voltaren pills, an anti-inflammatory drug. He's not supposed to take more than one a day, but he can't get through the day without at least three or four times the recommended dose. Possible side-effects: high blood pressure, heart failure, kidney problems, liver disease.

* * *

By the time we see the rheumatologist, we are desperate. She's a middle-aged woman with frizzy hair, flowy clothes, and a frazzled manner. But she takes an extremely thorough health history that starts in infancy, and I'm hopeful that this means she will get to the bottom of this. At some point she asks me to leave the room for the physical examination. I protest and say that Richard doesn't mind me staying, but no luck; I'm being unceremoniously kicked out.

I ask him afterwards what that was all about, and he says that she wanted to know about any possible STDs and sexual partners I may not know about to rule out Chlamydia. At this point we both wouldn't mind a touch of Chlamydia if that meant he would get better. Sadly, no Chlamydia for us.

It's not arthritis either. The doctor is now investigating for lupus, fibromyalgia, and multiple sclerosis.

The inflammation markers in his body are ten times as high as they should be, indicating that there is inflammation somewhere in his body, even if we haven't found the location yet.

Another Google-search reveals that it could also indicate cancer or an inflammation in the arteries of the heart, increasing his risk of a heart attack.

We are living in a nightmare. Richard is too weak to do chores by himself, so I do the heavy lifting for him. Every day before work I bring hay to the cows, sheep, and horses, and after work I carry the heavy buckets of feed to the birds, give more hay to the hay burners and feed the cats and dogs. Once it starts freezing, I also haul bucket after bucket of water to the animals. My arms are aching and I'm miserable; I'm not a fan of doing chores. But there's no way Richard can do it, and the animals need food and water.

When we are done, we collapse onto our respective couches in front of *Mad Men*, Richard swallowing strong pain pills like Skittles and me swallowing my own medicine – wine – right along Don Draper swigging his Old Fashioneds.

Richard has lost even more weight – thirty pounds in three months. Despite all the doctor's appointments, tests, and blood work we are no closer to a diagnosis.

One evening he says something that's chilling me to the bone. I am sitting on the floor next to the couch he's lying on, stroking his forehead, and murmuring something useless along the lines of "you will get better". I don't know that, but what else am I supposed to say?

With his eyes still closed he whispers: "Miriam, I can't go on like this much longer. I don't want to live like this if it doesn't get better."

My hand on his forehead stills. "What are you saying?"

"Just that. I don't know how much longer I can endure this." My entire body turns cold. Richard is the most life-loving person I know, and he's someone who *never* gives up. If he feels that he's reached the limit of how much pain and uncertainty he can endure it must mean that he's suffering even more than he lets on.

I want to stay strong, but this is too much. I murmur something about getting some fresh air and practically run outside, the dogs following in my wake. I instinctively head to the cows because they are very soothing. They have beautiful, soulful eyes, and even though it's dark and I can't see their eyes, listening to them chewing their food rhythmically is calming. I sink down in front of them and start crying quietly.

The dogs have settled down around me, licking my tears away and giving me all the comfort they can. I would be lost without them, that's for sure.

I stare into the darkness as hopelessness and fear are pressing down on me. We have both reached our limits, and I have absolutely no idea what to do. What will happen to us if we can't figure this out?

* * *

I haven't shared much of what's going on with others. A few friends know, but barely anybody else does. At work I pretend that everything is fine because I'm afraid that if I tell them how bad it is and how scared I am I will start screaming and never stop.

But now that things are in crisis mode, I confide in a few more people in hopes of getting that vital piece of information that will help us.

A co-worker suggests food allergies. "Try to go dairy-, gluten-, and sugar-free," is her advice. All Richard can stomach are those canned peaches, so that advice is not practical at the moment. I'm not a fan of food restriction and I don't have the energy to figure out such a restrictive eating plan. Besides, deep down I'm sure that this is not a food allergy he suddenly developed at age 63.

We keep returning to our doctor, hoping for answers, but he's as much at a loss as we are.

He prescribes prednisone and a different pain medication, and we continue to drag ourselves through our days, each in our individual version of hell: Richard in constant terrible joint, bone, and muscle pain, having fevers, chills, nausea, insomnia, fatigue, no appetite, brain fog, memory lapses, difficulty thinking, stabbing and burning pain throughout his body, dizziness, swollen lymph nodes, severe depression.

I go almost mad with worry and the agony of seeing the person I love most in the world suffer so horrendously and not being able to help him. I also don't sleep well and I'm permanently exhausted, having to juggle work and the farm, and carrying the fear that if we don't figure out what's wrong, the very worst could happen.

At night we lie on our couches, both trying to numb our pain, and hoping for a few hours of escapism by immersing ourselves into the world of advertising in 1960s New York.

Things are looking bleak.

But then I do something stupid – and it saves us.

Lyme Disease

"What's that smell?" Richard asks me a few days later. I've noticed it too and it gives me an ominous feeling in the pit of my stomach. It's a sickly-sweet smell, like something is rotting. At first I think it's a piece of garbage that the dogs dropped somewhere, but I can' find anything. Besides, the smell seems to follow me. If you've ever stepped in dog poop and were the last to notice you know how cringe-inducing it is.

I also have the nagging feeling that I forgot something important, but I can't remember what it is.

He comes closer and sniffs me. "It's coming from you," he says with conviction.

"You're right," I agree miserably. "But I'm not sick, I feel fine. What could it be?" I think hard about what the smell reminds me of. I know I've smelled it before, but where?

And then it comes to me; it smells like cellulitis. I'm not talking about the cute dimples most women have on their thighs and butt that the diet industry wants us to spend thousands of dollars on to get rid of, which is not only impossible but also completely unnecessary. That cellulitis is harmless and perfectly natural.

No, I'm talking about the other cellulitis, the truly bad one. Cellulitis in a medical sense is a bacterial skin infection that causes redness, swelling and pain and has a distinct odour. If untreated it can cause serious health problems such as permanent swelling of the affected limb or, in extreme cases, necrotizing fasciitis which is a deep-layer infection and can result in amputation or death.

Occasionally I encounter cellulitis in my job, which is always a great opportunity to practice my professional poker face by not cringing. Let me tell you, wearing a mask is a real blessing in those instances.

That's the smell I'm drenched in, but I can't have cellulitis, can I? I tear off my clothes and inspect every inch of my naked body in the full-length mirror. To me relief I can't find any telltale redness, just my harmless dimples. I blow them a kiss and get dressed again.

While it's a relief that I don't have a serious skin infection it still doesn't explain the cause of the stench.

I rack my brain for what else it could be while I'm gazing around the bathroom. And then a suspicion comes to me. *Shit.*

I had my period last week. Could I have forgotten a tampon inside myself? I whip down my pants again and start searching around down there for the string.

I can't find it.

"Rich!" I yell. "Come in here!" In my panic I momentarily forget about his difficulty to move, and when he doesn't appear I hop into the living room with my pants around my ankles.

"What's going on?" he asks.

"You have to check if I forgot a tampon inside."

The beauty of being married for a long time is that you've seen every inch of your partner inside and out. Richard doesn't flinch. "Okay."

I plop myself down on the floor, brace my feet against the couch he's lying on and lift my pelvis up in the air.

"I need my glasses," he says, and I swear, get up and grab a pair before repeating the maneuver.

Richard does some digging and comes up empty.

"The smell is definitely coming from there," he informs me, as if I don't know it myself. You'd have to be nose-blind not to notice it.

"What am I gonna do?" I shriek hysterically.

"You have to go to the hospital and get it taken out."

"I don't want to," I moan like a petulant five-year old.

"You *have* to," he empathizes. "This is dangerous, you could die of an infection."

Way to sugar-coat it, babe.

I know he's right, so I reluctantly agree. I get dressed again for the third time this morning and then I call my hospital to find out which doctor is on. There's no way in hell I'm gonna go there if it's someone I know well.

Sure enough, it's my favourite doctor whom I've worked with dozens of times. I have no doubt that he would be perfectly professional, but this is a hard no for me. Boundaries are important.

"I'm going to Kamloops," I announce, and that's exactly what I do.

During the one-hour drive to the hospital I try to retrace my steps. My period ended a week ago and I'm still not sure that I left a tampon in, but it's impossible to recall. There are so many thousands of little things we do automatically every day without thinking, and this is one of them. Besides, I'm pretty distracted these days, and most nights I've had a few glasses of wine. It's easy to lose track of things.

Three hours later the male, but thankfully unknown doctor pulls something out of me that can only be described as looking like a dead, decomposing mouse. I know because I make the mistake of glancing down upon hearing the doctor exclaim "aha, got it!"

I am very embarrassed and very relieved.

Once the doctor has left (which he does quickly, and who can blame him) I confess to the nurse how embarrassed I am.

"It happens several times a week," she reassures me, and whether it's true or not, I'm grateful for her kindness. Armed with a prescription for two different antibiotics I'm dismissed, feeling foolish yet grateful that my problem could be resolved that easily. If only the diagnosis for Richard's mystery illness would be as straightforward.

***

I decide to share this mishap on my blog. My process for writing is to put down whatever feels right. I share what's important to me, what I consider to be funny or interesting or useful to others. I figure my unfortunate event could help another woman, if only to let her know that this is apparently very common.

As an explanation for my absentmindedness, I mention Richard's health problems. I don't go into detail, just give a quick overview.

This turns out to be the most important blog post I have ever written.

A reader leaves this comment:

"*Mystery illnesses are not any fun! After a year of tests and specialists I was diagnosed with Lyme disease. The roving joint pain was a symptom. Just thought I would mention that. Best of luck getting to the bottom of it!*"

Reading her words sends a jolt of adrenaline through my body. Lyme disease? We haven't thought of that. I barely know what it is, and I've never googled anything so fast in my life.

I click on the website[1] and start reading. I don't want to get my hopes up in case it's just another dead end, but I can't help myself; I'm hopeful anyway.

That hope increases exponentially as I get to the list of symptoms: bone pain, joint pain and swelling, tennis elbow, stiff neck, muscle pain. It lists ringing in ears, oversensitivity to light, night sweats, unexplained chills, extreme fatigue, shortness of breath.

There are mood swings, unusual depression, insomnia, sleep apnea, memory loss.

And the clinchers: unexplained fevers, pain migrates to different body parts, continual [sinus] infections, increased effect from alcohol and worse hangovers.

My heart is beating fast now. This is it! This *must* be it! Richard has every single one of these symptoms! I speed-dial our doctor's office and make an urgent appointment for the next day. I know next to nothing about Lyme disease, so I settle in and continue reading.

Lyme Disease is an inflammatory disorder that is spread to humans through tick bites. Ticks pick up the bacteria through infected animals like deer, mice, or birds, and pass it on to whoever is unlucky enough to get bitten next. Some people get the telltale bulls-eye rash, but many don't.

---

[1] Canadian Lyme Disease Foundation, www.canlyme.com

It is dubbed "the mystery disease" due to the difficulty to diagnose it. There are more than one hundred symptoms associated with Lyme disease, which may or may not show up immediately. In many cases, patients won't have any symptoms for months or even years. If you are bitten by a nymph tick you may never know it; they are the size of this period →.

Blood tests often come back with false negatives, particularly in the early stages of the disease. The reason for this is that the bacteria don't circulate in the blood but interact directly with the cell tissue they infect, making it difficult to detect. They also replicate slowly, meaning the number of bacteria found in the patient stays small.

The blood test is looking for antibodies in the blood, and they need time to develop.

To make matters even worse, there is no universally accepted test for Lyme disease; Lyme tests in Canada are largely flawed.

Due to the difficulty of making a diagnosis, some people with diagnoses of rheumatoid arthritis, fibromyalgia, lupus, multiple sclerosis, or being accused of being hypochondriacs may in fact have Lyme Disease.

Reading all this doesn't discourage me. On the contrary, it makes me more convinced than ever that this is Richard's disease.

He can't remember being bitten by a tick, but that doesn't mean he wasn't. Many people don't get a rash, and if the tick falls off before it's engorged you'll never know you had an unwelcome passenger on board for a short while. Their bite is usually painless, and since they're so tiny in the nymph stage it's easy to not notice them. There are ticks in every place Richard has ever lived, so it could have happened anywhere.

When he had the same symptoms as a child in the 1960s, Lyme disease hadn't been discovered yet. It wasn't until 1982 that the American medical entomologist Willi Burgdorfer found the bacteria that cause Lyme disease, which had been an unknown affliction until then, thought to be caused by a virus.

I'm so impatient to see the doctor that I can't sleep. As soon as he steps into the room the next day I burst out: "I think Richard has Lyme disease!"

He looks thoughtful. "That could be it," he agrees and orders the standard two-tiered testing: the enzyme-linked immunosorbent assay (ELISA) test and the western blot test. ELISA measures the antibody response to the infection and comes back positive, meaning there are harmful antigens in his body that the antibodies are trying to fight off.

The western blot test is a bioanalytical method in which antibodies specific to the Borrelia burgdorferi antigens are visualized. It is more sensitive than the ELISA test and it comes back negative, but our doctor isn't concerned about that. "Late-stage antibody testing is much less accurate," he explains. "But based on your clinical symptoms and the positive ELISA test, let's start you on antibiotics and see if it helps."

He gives Richard a prescription for a month's worth of Doxycycline, tells us to keep him updated and sends us home. The effect is almost instantaneous. On day two of taking the antibiotics Richard's starting to feel better for the first time in four months. With each passing day he improves more. The brain fog is lifting, he's finding his words again, and his short- term memory is coming back with bells on. In fact, it's better than it has been in years. We suspect that the dormant Lyme bacteria in his body have been sneakily affecting his brain for years, if not decades.

It's the best Christmas present of our lives. After months of darkness, we can finally see the light again.

In January, Richard continues to improve, but not without setbacks. He's still in quite a lot of pain which has migrated from his lower body into his upper body, particularly his shoulders. It's a nasty, intense pain that keeps him white-faced and breathless and still unable to drive or lift anything heavier than a teacup. Sometimes it travels down his arms into his hands, or it likes to hang out below his collar bone in his pectoral muscle. The pain is making it impossible for him to sleep, which in turn means he's tired and fatigued almost all the time.

But towards the end of the month, we're going out for sushi for the first time in months. That's huge! Sushi dates are a stable of our relationship and adding that beloved routine back into our lives means we are one step closer to our normal life again.

In February, we return to our local pub for the first time in six months.

Everybody is pleased to see us, but they can't hide their shock at Richard's gaunt appearance.

"Is he okay?" I get asked more than once, and I assure them that yes, he's okay and much better than he was. I'm so used to the changes since I'm around him every day that I don't notice it anymore, but now that I'm looking at him from across the room, I see what everybody else sees: a frail man who moves cautiously, as if afraid to fall. He looks like one of the soldiers portrayed on TV who return home after having seen and done horrible things in war and who are sleepwalking through their old life, feeling dazed and out of place.

In a way, he has been through a war. He has endured terrible pain, insomnia, stress, and fear for his life. No wonder he looks shell-shocked.

In March, Richard can reach his left ear with his left hand again. He is also able to grind a pepper mill, lift a bucket with feed, and best of all – drive! He drives two hours each way to visit a friend and feels like he ran a marathon afterwards: exhausted and in pain but proud.

With the arrival of spring our life gets busier, which in turn makes Richard sicker again. His weakened body needs plenty of rest, and if there's too much activity going on, even something as fun as having friends over, he gets sore and exhausted. His short-term memory has declined again, his constant shoulder pain is back more severely than it has been in a while, and his energy levels are very low.

His recovery is one step forward and two back, but we are slowly figuring out what works and what doesn't. Plenty of rest is what he needs most, so I'm still doing morning chores while he stays in bed until noon. He goes outside for a few hours in the afternoon, but sometimes he will have to take a break and rest for a while. After dinner he always lies down and usually falls asleep quickly.

* * *

After six straight months of taking antibiotics twice a day Richard is almost back to normal. He barely needs any anti-inflammatory or pain medication anymore because he can handle his post-treatment Lyme disease syndrome with rest and a tranquil lifestyle.

Richard is feeling fine again – but I'm more traumatized than I realize at the time.

The effects of the months of stress and worry will continue to create unpleasant ripples in my life for years to come.

Depression

I should be on top of the world. Richard has mostly recovered his health, we've built my dream She Shed with the wrap-around porch I always wanted, and my first book comes out. The support I receive for it from my old and new work families is overwhelming. There is a potluck and book signing at my old hospital in Langley where I reconnect with people whom I haven't seen in months or years, but who showed up to buy a copy and tell me how proud they are. It's impossible to adequately express how much this means to me; saying thank you doesn't even begin to do cover it, but that's all I have. In a moment of recklessness, I ask the manager of the hospital gift shop if they would sell my book, and they say yes! I'm thrilled.

Buoyed by my success in Langley I screw up my courage, approach a local business in town and ask if they would consider stocking my book. They agree as well. I'm on a roll! I'm also red-faced and stammering with nerves, and I feel deeply embarrassed without being able to say what for.

But that's only the beginning. The staff at my work gets wind of my book and they really come through: they *all* want to buy it from me. And not only do they buy it they also read it and then come to me and tell me how much they loved it. I'm touched by the kindness of my co-workers whom I've only known for a little over a year and who treat me as one of their own.

A few times I get recognized at work by patients who've read the book and tell me how much they enjoyed it. I'm x-raying someone while they're telling me how much my story resonated with them, which is one of the more surreal experiences of my life.

Another day when I come to work, I see a patient sitting in the waiting room, reading my book, and my first impulse is to run and hide. What is wrong with me? I'm so happy and overjoyed to see this. I'm on this wild ride that I've been fantasizing about for so long, and you would think that I'm flying high.

But for some reason I can barely stand the attention. As much as I want to enjoy it, I'm not feeling worthy of it. I'm afraid that any moment someone will march up to me and tell me that I'm a fraud.

At night I soothe my jangled nerves with several glasses of wine, the signature drink of tortured writers everywhere. Maybe if I drink enough, I'll start to believe that I'm one of them?

The thing about fulfilling my dream is that I assumed it would come with improved self-esteem, maybe even a little swagger of confidence. I naively hoped that I would magically become the confident, calm, and strong woman I've always yearned to be. With everything going right in my life it was the logical next step, wasn't it?

Instead I'm feeling as fragile and raw as a freshly hatched bird, and I just can't figure out why.

* * *

Then Kate Spade and Anthony Bourdain kill themselves within days of each other – and I suddenly understand. *Fuuuuuck.* My depression is back.

Their deaths hit me deeply. They were both heroes in their respective fields: highly successful, beloved, creative, charismatic people. And yet, the demons in their heads won in the end, and every time mental illness wins it results in a terrible loss for all of us.

I stay in bed all weekend, unable to get up. I'm grieving like I knew them personally: crying, eating ice cream, feeling hopeless. I'm also terrified because a small part of me understands why they did it.

I re-read Bourdain's book *Kitchen Confidential*, searching for clues. Did he have any inkling when he wrote it that he would lose his battle one day?

I scour the Internet for details about their lives, trying to avoid the comments about their deaths. I know what people who have no idea what it's like living with depression say about someone who commits suicide:

"*How can they be so selfish?*"

"*What about their children?*"

"*They had everything, what did they have to be depressed about?*"

"*If they knew how much they meant to us, they wouldn't have done it.*"

"*How could they do this to me?*"

I'm in the unenviable position of having first-hand experience with depression, so let me enlighten you.

Mental illness is a disease of the brain. The brain is the organ that controls thought, memory, emotion, and dozens of other important processes in the body – it's the organ that makes us who we are.

The heinousness of mental illness is that the organ that's sick is in charge of making decisions. It's a recipe for disaster, like putting a tantrum-prone toddler in charge of his family and then being surprised that he makes them eat cookies for dinner and draw on the walls. Is it rational? Of course not. He is two years old. His developing brain isn't yet able to make rational decisions. My brain during a depressive episode is like that of a two-year old toddler. It does the best it can with what it has but it is not rational.

Let me describe a depressive episode to you:

It starts with a loss of colour. It happens gradually so you don't notice it at first, until you're suddenly hit by how grey everything looks around you. In your inner landscape the birds have stopped singing, the sun has disappeared, and an icy wind has picked up. A storm is coming, and you desperately search for shelter, trying to stay dry; but you already know it's impossible. You are about to get drenched, and the only question that remains is how long you'll have to stay wet.

While you try to wait out the storm, soaked and shivering, your depression buzzes around your brain like a thousand mosquitos, tormenting you with your worst fears.

Nobody loves you.

Everybody finds you annoying.

You will never be happy again.

You are a burden.

Your sick brain is twisting everything wonderful in your life into something terrible. All the things you normally love to do don't give you joy anymore. Not only that, but your brain is also telling you that *they never gave you any joy in the first place.* **Everything in your life has been a lie.**

And there is a small but insistent mosquito buzzing into your ear: wouldn't the world be better off without you?

Here's the kicker: while all this is happening in your mind you might look quite normal on the outside. You may miss a day of work, but often you don't. You gather all your strength, put on your mask, and venture out into the world, acting like everything is fine.

We are hiding our mental illness as a self-defence mechanism because of how the world reacts to invisible illness.

Despite some progress being made, our society still struggles to accept invisible illnesses as being real, because you can't prove what you can't see.

Is she really depressed or is she an attention-seeking drama queen?

Can't she get up or does she not *want* to get up because she's lazy?

I've had someone say to me: "I want to stay in bed all day too, but I don't do it because I'm an adult and I have responsibilities." Translation: I'm better than you.

Many people seem to believe that depression is a choice, and if we really wanted to, we could snap out of it. Other people act like it's our fault when we have a mental illness because of bad choices we have made in life. This can be anything: dropping out of school, cheating, getting into debt, becoming homeless, being on drugs, betraying our friends, becoming estranged from our families, or a thousand other things. It depends on what the person making the judgment deems as unacceptable. Never mind that the cause behind these behaviours often *is* mental illness and that it's not necessarily a person's free decision to act the way they do, but a result of being mentally ill.

Another stigma around mental illness is the ridiculous yet prevalent assumption that successful or rich people should not be depressed because they have no reason. Reminder: mental illness is not a choice. It's just as absurd as saying that successful or rich people shouldn't get cancer, and if they do it's selfish. Or that some (poor, disadvantaged, uneducated) people deserve it more than others.

* * *

Eventually the storm passes, and the sun come out again. You get dry and warm and comfy. The world is bright and colourful again, filled with birdsong, beauty, and joy. Sometimes that phase lasts a long time, weeks or even months. In fact, you may get so comfortable that you begin to think that your depression is gone forever. All the good stuff you are doing for your mental health is paying off, and maybe you're cured?

The danger with that thinking is the temptation to quit taking your meds. I've been on antidepressants since late 2012, and when I first started taking them and experienced the sweet relief that you get when your neurotransmitters are balanced, I was sure I would never go back.

But a few years pass, and you get complacent. You've read somewhere that meditation is better than any medication, and I meditate once in a while. Your hippie friend encourages you to ask yourself "what depresses you?", to find an answer to that question and remove the depressant. Problem solved. You start to wonder if maybe you overreacted all those times you thought you were depressed – maybe it's not that bad? After all, that's the message you hear all the time, and maybe all those people know something you don't.

It's bullshit and it's dangerous. I've tried to wean myself off my antidepressants, and it wasn't pretty. The reason why I feel good most of the time is *because* of the medication. Glennon Doyle puts it perfectly in her brilliant book *Untamed*:

"Going off meds because you feel better is like standing in a torrential rainstorm holding a trusty umbrella that is keeping you dry and thinking: Wow. I'm so dry. It's probably time to get rid of this silly umbrella.

Stay dry and alive."

* * *

That's my frame of mind in June 2018: I'm depressed; I feel guilty about not being over the moon about the release and surrounding support of my book; I feel even guiltier for being down when Richard is mostly healthy again, and I should be beyond thrilled and grateful. Life is good – but all I want to do is hide.

I can barely make it out of bed for a week. One of the worst things about being in a depression is the overwhelming exhaustion and bone-tiredness. It's paralyzing. It can take half an hour before you can make yourself get out of bed to pee. You will notice that you need to pee, and you tell your body to get up. But your body acts like it's super-glued to your mattress. You lie there, staring at the ceiling, trying to be firmer. *Get up now, body, the bathroom is right next door! It's twelve steps away.* But you remain motionless. *This is ridiculous* you think to yourself, but it doesn't make a lick of difference. You continue to have this fruitless conversation with yourself, feeling more and more disgusted with your own uselessness.

Only the threat of peeing your bed will eventually give you enough strength to muster the superhuman effort it requires to heave your body out of bed and drag it to the bathroom. Your body feels like it's made of cement and weighs a thousand pounds. You avoid looking in the mirror because you know that you look like death warmed over. Before you retrace the twelve steps back to bed you venture into the kitchen for supplies: junk food and wine.

Oh yes, baby: it's time to self-medicate.

Depression and Alcohol

The thing about depression is that your mind is a real asshole. The voices inside your head keep up a running commentary about what a waste of space you are, and with non-existent confidence that's hard to take. You believe everything they say, because you can't see things objectively thanks to your faulty brain. Rationality has left the building, and you are stuck with these hooligans who have taken over your thinking, feeling, and being. You are under constant attack physically, mentally, and emotionally, and it is agony. Imagine being tied to a chair, and every person you are afraid of, has hurt you or made fun of you is standing right in front of you, free to say whatever the hell they want. All the bullies you've ever encountered in your life have joined forces and are hurling insults at you while you sit there helplessly, begging them to stop, but knowing full well they won't until they've reduced you to a quivering, beaten down heap.

The dementors in J.K. Rowling's *Harry Potter* are a metaphor for depression based on her own experience with the disease. Different characters throughout the books describe what it feels like to be close to them, and the descriptions are perfect: they talk about the happiness being sucked out of them, which makes them feel like they will never be cheerful again. They report a bone-chilling cold, a hopelessness that settles over them, and the absolute conviction that nothing good will ever happen again. As long as someone is near dementors, they are forced to relive the worst experiences of their life over and over.

Anyone with depression knows how accurate these descriptions are. The pain and suffering are as real as if you broke your leg. That's why some people who are depressed self-harm – the physical pain eases the mental one.

How do you shut the voices up? Deep down I know that this will pass. I've been in this storm often enough to know that if I just hang on, if I find shelter where I can wait it out, the storm will eventually exhaust itself and die away. But getting through it is the hard part, and I'm at my most vulnerable when I'm being tied to that chair in front of my enemies. What to do? How to lessen the pain?

I've found an imperfect solution: distraction and drinking. Distraction is a no-brainer: anything that helps me mute the bullies in my head is welcome. TV shows are an obvious choice, as long as they are easy to follow, entertaining, and ideally contain a fair amount of flawed people. Heavy drinking, drug use, maybe a sex addiction or shoplifting habit are appreciated, so I feel better about myself in comparison. That's why *Mad Men* was such a good show to watch while Richard was sick and I slowly lost my mind – in comparison to Don and Betty Draper's dysfunctional marriage, constant smoking, and insane alcohol consumption, we were doing alright. I also like to re-watch shows I've seen a gazillion times before, because their predictability is comforting. Another reason why it's beneficial to watch shows I've seen before is because I'm usually on my phone while I watch *and* drink wine at the same time, and it's tricky to follow a plot with this double whammy of distractions.

Before you're impressed by my multitasking talents, it's important to note that I barely take anything in. If I use D&D (distraction and drinking) for self-medication purposes, I will *not* retain anything I see, read, watch, or listen to. All it does is drown out the destructive noise in my head and make me numb. If I'm lucky I'll have the illusion along the way that I'm feeling cheered up, even if it isn't real. But mostly it's the slow building of a soundproof wall between me and my own thoughts – a self-defence mechanism that's supposed to protect me.

You've probably already detected the problem with this approach: the soundproof wall doesn't discriminate. It doesn't keep the bad thoughts out and lets the happy thoughts through. Nope, once you build the wall you separate yourself from all feelings, good and bad. What you are left with is a vacuum devoid of emotions. It's not a nice place to be.

People often mistakenly think that being depressed means being sad. That's wrong. Being sad is a healthy and necessary emotion. If something painful has happened to you or you have lost something or someone important, sadness tells you that you need extra care and compassion from yourself and others. It's not a sign of weakness, it's one of our strongest emotions. Evolutionary, sadness is meant to be displayed in a way that others notice and react to. Since humans don't have natural defenses like claws or venom, our ability to co-exist in a group is our greatest strength. Our automatic response to the sadness of another human being is to comfort them. This empathy regulates the nervous system of the sad person, which in turn engages the thinking brain. Thinking and applying logic is our secret weapon that has allowed us to grow and evolve.

Depression is very different from sadness. Its worst characteristic is that you feel dead inside. Nothing gives you pleasure; you can't remember *ever* having felt pleasure in your life. Life just seems to be a never-ending stretch of grey, joyless days. You can't figure out what the purpose of it is. What are you even doing here? Everything seems utterly pointless. You may have silenced the mean voices in your brain, but you've silenced the kind ones as well. All you're left with is a big, fat nothing.

While your insides are dead, your outsides are often hurting. Depression presents with physical symptoms as well as mental ones. For me it's severe exhaustion and aches all over my body. It feels like the beginnings of a flu but without the sympathy of others. Everybody feels sorry for you when you have the flu; nobody does when you can't get out of bed because of depression.

The other big difference to sadness is that you will hide your depression. The care and comfort we receive from others when we are sad helps us to feel better. But depression usually doesn't show up without shame, and shame prompts us to hide our condition. If we have to call in sick to work, we feign a stomach bug, a cold, or menstrual cramps.

If we manage to drag our sorry selves to work, we slap on a forced smile and avoid conversation. There's no room for small talk or idle chitchat – we need every ounce of energy we can scrape together just to make it through the day.

It's staggeringly exhausting and will leave us with a completely empty tank. The smallest thing after a day that cost you all your energy reserves will push you over the edge – bad traffic, a child or spouse wanting attention, seeing dirty cups piled next to the dishwasher instead of stacked inside it. Forget about dinner or a cozy chat about your day – we are done.

Living like this is terrible. That's why I pour myself a large glass of wine as soon as I come home and turn to Netflix to drown out my reality.

I know that it would be better for me if I would do some yoga or meditation, but I have no strength in me to do anything but Savasana, the aptly named corpse pose, and they don't call it the hardest pose for nothing – I have zero relaxation in me. And meditation in my state? Are you kidding? The voices in my head would kill me.

Nope, the slow buzz and numbing of booze is just what the doctor ordered. Well, my doctor doesn't exactly know that I'm mixing my antidepressants with alcohol, but he's also never told me not to do it. What he doesn't know can't hurt him, right? If it can hurt me is another question, but one I'm not asking myself right now.

The first sip provides instant relief. For a moment I feel a tiny bit of hope as the dopamine rush hits my brain. But that feeling doesn't last. The initial happy tipsiness is soon replaced by drunkenness that during a depressive episode makes me sometimes angry, but usually weepy.

I don't realize yet how much worse alcohol makes depression and anxiety; I will talk more about that in chapter 22.

All I know right now is that I wake up at 2 am, my personal witching hour, filled with shame and regret. I have terrible "hanxiety", anxiety that is caused by a hangover and gives you existential dread, nonstop worrying and a crushing sense of self-loathing. That's a lot to deal with at two in the morning, especially when you already feel more fragile than usual.

The feeling of shame is especially excruciating. Dr. Brené Brown, who has done extensive research on shame and vulnerability, says this: "*I define shame as the intensely painful feeling or experience of believing that we are flawed and therefore unworthy of love and belonging – something we've experienced, done, or failed to do makes us unworthy of connection."*[2]

If you've ever woken up in the middle of the night you know that problems look about a hundred times worse than they really are. You may also be familiar with the entirely unhelpful habit of replaying every painful or embarrassing thing you've ever done in your life, no matter if it happened yesterday or twenty years ago. I have no control over the worrying, self-hate, or reel in my head that plays *The Worst Moments of Miriam* on a loop. It's my private hell, and there's only one way how I can get through it: by turning to my great love.

I switch on the light and reach for my Kindle on the nightstand. Words are the saviours that help me escape my bleak reality. I read until my eyelids droop, and I fall asleep, often with the light on and the eBook resting gently on my chest.

* * *

This depression is so bad that I'm desperate enough to go to my family doctor for help. I start crying as soon as I sit down in his office, which is awkward because we work together, and he only knows me as cheerful and upbeat. He offers to increase my dose of antidepressants, which is not really what I want. I clumsily ask about counselling, and he agrees that this might be helpful, but when I ask him how to find a counsellor he suggests looking up the local family counselling office and giving them a call. I don't have the courage to ask him for a referral, or to find out if I even need one, so I just nod and whisper "okay, thanks".

I leave with a prescription for more happy pills, feeling defeated.

Shortly after that visit I come across a job posting that catches my attention. It's for a job out of town, one week on/one week off, and it would require me to stay there a week at a time because of being on call after my shift. While I would ordinarily never consider a job where I'm away from home 50% of the time, now I'm intrigued. Running away from the attention to a place where

---

[2] Brené Brown: Shame vs. Guilt, https://brenebrown.com/articles/2013/01/15/shame-v-guilt

nobody knows that I wrote a book is incredibly appealing. It would also mean regular hours and more money, because right now my only employment is on a casual basis with no guaranteed hours. And then there's a secret reason I don't even admit to myself: I need a reason not to drink wine almost every night, and I don't drink when I'm on call.

On my next day off I drive to the town to check it out. It's an 80-minute drive through woods, gently rolling hills, past sparkling lakes and sprawling ranches, and when I drive by a big field I see a herd of deer grazing peacefully, their fawns running around and playing happily. The picturesque drive makes me exhale for the first time in weeks.

The town is small and quaint with a few cute cafés and restaurants, an adorable gift shop, and a pretty town centre. The hospital is surrounded by trees, the lawns in front of it are dotted with benches and a little pavilion that looks perfect for eating lunch, and – would you believe it? There is a deer with her fawn standing in the plant bed right next to the entrance!

Inside I get a quick tour from the technologist who's working that day, and afterwards I stroll around the premises, thinking. I'm calmer than I have been in a long time. This feels right.

I discuss the job with Richard. He leaves the decision up to me, assuring me that he will support me no matter what I decide. He's seen that I'm struggling, but even he doesn't know the full extent of how bad it is.

The shame of depression is so severe that I've never been able to tell him the worst of it. One reason is that I can't properly put it into words; but the other, more important one is that I don't want anybody to see the darkest, ugliest part of me. It's not only the depression I'm ashamed of – the worst secret I'm keeping is my self-medication of it. Richard doesn't know just how much I drink to drown out the voices and stop my brain from overthinking, because I'm very careful about hiding it.

More days than not I drink a bottle a night. There just doesn't seem to be a good enough reason not to do it. The way I pour it's only three glasses, and that's not really that much, is it? The French have been drinking buckets of wine for centuries, and they have one of the longest life expectancies off all the developed countries.

And everybody does it, don't they? It's what I see all around me on TV, social media, in commercials, stores, and printed on T-shirts.

"I only drink wine on days that end with a 'y'."

"Age and glasses of wine should never be counted."

"Wine is the answer, but I can't remember the question."

"Wine a little and you'll feel better."

And good old Ernest Hemingway: "My only regret in life is that I did not drink more wine."

We joke about it at work, chuckling at the co-worker's mug that says, "I wish this were wine". There's no social gathering, book club, party, or girl's night without booze. All our friends drink, and we drink every time we hang out. It's everywhere, and I tell myself there are worse habits. I don't smoke or do any drugs, I eat healthyish, and I move my body regularly. We live in an area with plenty of fresh, healthy country air, and we have no major stress in our life – if you disregard Richard's near-death experience the previous year, my less-than-ideal mental health, and typical adult life stuff.

Besides, I don't drink every day. There are regular nights where I (force myself to) abstain, pretending that I'm fine while secretly pining for a glass of wine.

I *never* drink when I'm on call, but I'm rarely on call more than a handful of nights a month. Being on call seven days in a row, two weeks out of the month would be a game changer, and some instinct tells me that it's important that I go for it.

I accept the job. It starts in August, just a few weeks from now, and amid the turmoil of erratic and conflicting feelings a new emotion is starting to sprout their first, fragile buds: excitement.

What's the saying: a change is as good as a rest? I'm about to find out if there is any truth to it.

Going Away

I wake up and pull the dogs close, showering them with kisses and hugging them a little bit too hard.

I also hug Richard a little bit too hard until he gently pushes me away and tells me: "Dragging it out won't make it any easier. You have to go now." He is right of course, but when I turn away for the final time, I have to take several deep breaths to prevent myself from crying. I lift my blue suitcase into my trunk, give my corgi Lily a last kiss on the nose, and then I start the car. I slowly make my way up the driveway, watching the foals gallop around the field, tails up in the air and loving life. I fill up the goats' water bucket, wave goodbye to them and then I'm off. It's 5:45 in the morning.

I hate goodbyes. Who doesn't? Since I moved from Germany to Canada at the age of 23, I've had more than my fair share of goodbyes. The nature of moving away from your first family to create your second is that you will always have to leave someone you love. But leaving Richard is by far the hardest for me. He's my North Star, my port in the storm, my best friend in the world. At this moment I can't imagine what I was thinking. Why am I doing this? My heart is heavy, and I have a little cry in the car. Crying gets a bad rep, but I love it. It's scientifically proven that it's self-soothing because it activates the parasympathetic nervous system, it relieves stress, and it releases endorphins that make you feel better. Sure enough, I feel calmer after a few minutes. I dry my eyes and settle in to enjoy the drive.

The rising sun is blood-red, struggling to make her way through the smoke in the air. The forest fires are upon us, and smoke is wafting all around the Interior of British Columbia. It creates an eerie atmosphere that's half end-times, half fantasy land. Anything seems possible: dinosaurs may step out of the forest, or maybe zombies or medieval knights – none of them would look out of place. Frodo Baggins and his fellow hobbits would be right at home in this landscape on their quest to destroy the ring; or is all this smoke caused by Daenerys Targaryen's dragons?

Driving through nature is one of life's great pleasures. I can't believe I haven't done more of it lately. But when you work where you live and have everything you need close by, your world gets smaller. Your range of daily movement dwindles to where you have to go, which for me is about fifteen kilometers. I haven't been aware of it, but since Richard's illness my world has shrunk to what's contained within those fifteen kilometers. That's insane! Just last year we would drive 200 kilometers each way just to meet our friends for dinner, and this year I've barely left the confines of home, work, local pub, and the stores in town. I can't believe I didn't notice it before.

I think it was Isaac Newton who figured out that a body in motion stays in motion, and a body at rest stays at rest, and he was right about that. I've caged myself in mentally and have been at a standstill for months. Time to break down the barriers I've erected in my mind and expand my world again.

***

I arrive in town shortly past 7 o'clock. The main street is lined with leafy trees and old-fashioned lamp posts, each decorated with huge, overflowing flower baskets. A few dog walkers are out and about, but other than that the town is still quiet. I drive up to the hospital and park my car. Two deer stand just feet away, grazing peacefully, unperturbed by my presence. I smile at my friendly welcome committee and then I walk into my new place of work.

I'm nervous. As I step into the building I first notice the institutionalized wall colour, the fluorescent lights, and a sea of strange faces. My impulse is to run to my desk and then hide there for as long as possible, letting the people come to me. But I know that this is the surest way to stay the new girl, and I'm determined to make the most of this experience. I tell my introverted self to be brave, take a deep breath, and venture out.

I make the rounds through the building, introducing myself to every person I encounter. Without fail they greet me warmly with a smile, and my heart lifts. As soon as I'm back at my desk I write down all the new names of the people I've just met with a brief description, so I will learn them quicker.

The next day when I come in, I greet every person I see by name: the clerk, the lab techs and assistants I share the office with, the doctor on duty and the nurses I already met. I introduce myself to the ones I don't. And you know what? I notice the institutionalized wall colour less today.

When a co-worker asks me to come boxing with her that night, instead of saying no, I agree – *and then I even show up*. And just like that, there are two buildings in this new town that don't feel strange or intimidating anymore – the hospital and the gym. My new town has become more familiar already.

I'm staying at a hotel for the week but need to look for a more permanent accommodation. I make appointments to look at three rooms for rent and set out optimistically. The pictures of the first house have looked fantastic online: a gorgeous log home sitting on a hill bathed in sunshine. The reality is less glossy and filtered (real estate photos use more filters than the Kardashians), but no matter. I park my car in front of the somewhat shabby looking house and get out. A little girl of about eight is doing cartwheels and stops abruptly when she sees me.

"Who are you?" she challenges me, arms on non-existent hips.

I'm slightly taken aback. "I'm Miriam," I tell her and smile. She looks unimpressed. "Are you gonna live with us?" she asks.

"Maybe, I'm taking a look at the room now," I explain.

She has lost interest and resumes her cartwheels.

I head to the front door and ring the doorbell. An elderly man opens the door and invites me in. He looks – well, dirty is the only appropriate term. His clothes are stained, his rugged face is covered in white stubble, and the sparse hair on his head is stringy and filthy.

"Hello, hello!" he greets me enthusiastically and gives me a once-over. Behind him, two younger guys have appeared in the hallway, equally rough looking. One of them is only wearing shorts, his muscular, tattooed upper body looking like he acquired those muscles and tattoos in prison. The other one is openly checking me out and smiling broadly, not in a nice way. It's a hot August day and I'm wearing shorts and a sleeveless top, an outfit I regret now. These guys are giving me the creeps.

"H-hi," I stammer. "I'm here to take a look at the room?" I've already decided that there's no way in hell I will live here, but something – the innate female need to please and be polite, most likely – makes me play along. I figure I should at least act like I'm interested and pretend that everything is fine. The elderly man is the landlord and he's giving me the tour. He tells me that he and his wife live upstairs with their foster child Tabetha, the girl I met outside. I'm alarmed that this unkempt old man is looking after a little girl in a house where these unsettling guys live in the basement. I fervently hope that the wife has better hygiene and the temperament of a protective lion mama.

He's renting out four bedrooms on the ground floor. Three are already taken – all by guys who work at the mine – and the fourth one is available. There is a shared kitchen and two bathrooms, so two people have to share one bathroom. The two men who've loitered in the hallway have now moved to the kitchen, and they express their hope that I will join their happy little family. *When hell freezes over*, I think to myself, but aloud I simply say "maybe".

"You should meet my wife," the landlord tells me, and I agree, mostly for Tabetha's sake. I want to take a quick look at the woman who is caring for her to make sure there's one non-creepy adult in her life. There's no staircase leading from the ground to the first floor; you have to go outside, walk halfway around the house, and then enter through a separate entryway. Good for Tabetha, less ideal for the lone woman who moves in with three guys. This just reinforces my decision to get as far away from this place as possible. To my immense relief, the wife is a kind, motherly woman. She appears to be in her sixties, and she radiates the warmth of a beloved grandmother. That impression increases when she offers me iced tea and tells me that, should I take the room, I'm welcome any time to spend my evenings up here with them. I thank her profusely and tell them I will let them know my decision by the end of the day. I have no idea why I don't just say right then that I'm not going to take the room – that damn need not to offend rears its annoying head again.

As I'm leaving Tabetha stops her cartwheels again. "Are you gonna live with us?" she repeats her earlier question. I glance over my shoulder to make sure nobody is within earshot.

"No, I won't," I say gently. I don't want to lie to a child. She shrugs her shoulders as if she couldn't care less. "Okay bye." Okay bye, indeed. See you all never.

The second place is even worse. As I arrive the current occupant is in the process of moving out, and the lady who is showing me around (a friend of the landlord who lives out of town) is angrily whispering that the tenant should have moved out days ago. "I can't wait to see the back of her," she tells me conspiratorially and I force a smile. People like her gossip about everyone in their life, and I know that I wouldn't be an exception, no matter how well-behaved a tenant I would be. This is an apartment, not just a room, and it becomes clear right away why it is so cheap. The place is a dump. The baseboards are broken, walls dirty, the carpet is a health hazard, the blinds are ripped half off, and the sliding door to the shabby patio doesn't lock. "I'll get that fixed," she says, but it doesn't matter. I tell her thanks but no thanks and hightail it outta there.

When I tell my co-workers about that place the next day, the lab assistant looks at me in horror. "You went to *that* house?!" she exclaims in disbelief. "Druggies and criminals live there. I'd drag you out myself if you would have moved in. It's dangerous!"

* * *

You needed that context to understand why I say yes to option number three. What's behind door number three? Well, from the outside it looks nice. It's a neat house at the end of a quiet street with trees all around it. In the front window hang crystals and stained-glass ornaments. I'm cautiously optimistic as I ring the doorbell. A middle-aged woman opens the door with a German Shepherd by her side. My face lights up. The hardest part of being away from home is not having the dogs with me, so living in a house with a dog would be great!

"Hi, come right in. Ignore the dog, don't interact at all with her, okay?"

Uhm, what?

Bewildered, I follow the lady into her house. It's a nice space with pictures of horses *everywhere*. Uh-oh, am I in the presence of the special breed I like to call crazy horsewoman? Not every woman who owns and loves horses is a crazy horsewoman. There are many who are perfectly lovely people who simply happen to adore horses. To qualify as crazy horsewoman the following qualifications have to be present:

- Bossy
- Opinionated
- Permanently low on cash
- Love their horses more than their husbands, and probably
- their children
- Spend all of their money on horses
- Have an excuse for everything their horses do/don't do
- Decorate their houses lavishly with horse paraphernalia
- Are always covered in horsehair
- Can kick your ass, so you better watch out

Crazy horsewomen are to be approached with utter caution. Under normal circumstances I give them a wide berth because they scare the shit out of me. But these are not normal circumstances and I'm desperate. Am I desperate enough to live with one of them though? You are about to find out.

Linda invites me to have a seat in her living room. Already having forgotten her instruction to ignore the dog I make eye contact with her and try to coax her to me. The dog wags her tail and starts to approach me.

"NO!"

Dog and I both startle and look at Linda. She sternly points her outstretched hand towards a dog bed in the corner. "GO LAY DOWN ON YOUR BED!" she says firmly, and the dog tucks her tail in and slinks to her bed.

Linda looks at me reproachfully. "I told you not to interact with Belinda," she reprimands me.

"I'm so sorry, I forgot," I tell her sheepishly. I feel like a six-year-old who has been scolded by her mom for touching the stove.

Linda softens slightly. "Belinda is a rescue, and it's very important that she knows her boundaries," she explains. "If you interact with her, she gets wild, and I don't want that. When she's at home she's supposed to always stay on her bed. Please don't engage with her at all, okay?"

What? Did I hear that right that the dog is not allowed to move freely around the house? Yikes, that lady *is* crazy. I sneak another look at Belinda, and I swear she looks at me beseechingly as if to say, "see what I have to put up with?" I quickly look away. This is going to be hard, but it's her dog and her house.

"Okay," I mutter, filled with resentment. Great, I've now reverted to a sullen 16-year-old.

After the initial rocky introduction, we chat amicably for a few minutes. Linda somehow manages to pack a lot of her life story into a short amount of time, telling me about her divorce, her estranged daughter, her financial woes, and her horse. In case you're keeping track, Linda fully qualifies as crazy horsewoman. This doesn't bode well.

"Can I see the room?" I ask eventually when she draws breath.

"Oh yes, of course!" she laughs. We walk down a narrow, short hallway and she points out the closed door to one bedroom where another tenant lives. "Seo-Jun is from Korea," she tells me. "She works at the mine in the office. Nice girl, very quiet. She's at work right now."

She then indicates a door at the end of the hallway. "That's my bedroom."

Right next to it is the room she has available, possibly mine if I decide to take it. She opens it and steps back.

The first thing I see is the washer/dryer unit to the left. The next are the shelves along the right wall piled high with boxes, books, paper, kitchen gadgets, and Christmas decorations. A jolly Santa figurine waves at me. Along the only available wall she squeezed a single bed under the window with a nightstand next to it. The remaining floor space is barely big enough to fit a yoga mat next to the bed. The room is little more than a storage closet; a storage closet she wants $550 for. I'm momentarily speechless.

"I'll clean up the shelves if you decide to take it," she says after the silence between us becomes uncomfortable. "And I'd only do laundry during the week you are not here," she adds. I still haven't said a word. Is she for real?

"Uhm, I'll have to think about it," I finally tell her.

"I can lower the rent to $500 since you're only here two weeks a month?" she offers slightly desperately. I can't help but feel sorry for her. She's mentioned earlier that she only rents to women, and in a town with a mill and a mine, most people looking for a place are men.

"How about I can come back on the weekend with my husband? I'd like his opinion, and for you two to meet," I suggest, and she eagerly agrees.

My plan is to find something better, but this turns out to be impossible. There is nothing else available for rent unless I'm willing to pay over a thousand dollars, and I don't want to do that for two weeks a month. I go to three different motels in town and inquire about rates, but with hunting season rapidly approaching they're jacking their rates up and laugh me out the door when I ask about a deal. "We could probably do something in the winter," one of them offers half-heartedly, but that is of no help to me now.

When Richard arrives on Sunday, I take him to Linda. He's very knowledgeable about horses and the two of them have a good conversation going while I look around me and imagine myself living there. Seo-Jun is in the kitchen, cooking, and I wander over to meet her. She's a very nice young woman and we chat a bit about her work, Korea, and what it's like living here. "It's okay," she says noncommittally.

"How long have you lived here?" I ask, and she tells me six months. This gives me hope. If she's lasted that long then it can't be that bad, can it?

I ask Richard's opinion after we've left. "She's nuts, but harmless," is his verdict of Linda.

"But should I take it?" I press him.

"Babe, that's up to you. Why don't you try it out for a while? It's not like you have any other options right now."

He's right, of course. I text Linda and tell her that I'll move in on my next rotation. She's thrilled and reminds me to bring the $500 rent in cash. *It will be fine* I try to tell myself. Somehow, I don't quite believe myself.

* * *

I only last a week. I move in on a Thursday afternoon, and twenty-four hours later our relationship is done.

It starts off with the fact that the room looks exactly how it did when I last saw it, meaning all the stuff is still in there. She hasn't removed a single item despite her promise. But what really does it is how she treats Belinda. She reprimands that poor dog non-stop, and I can't bear it. When I come home on Friday after work Belinda greets me at the door, tail wagging, and I pet and hug her. She's a sweet dog, skittish and desperate for some attention, and I can't ignore her, I just can't. Linda isn't home so I figure it's safe – but I'm wrong. I've kept my door open, and Belinda is in my room when Linda comes home. To say she isn't pleased is an understatement. Linda goes ballistic. She yells at me, and she yells at the dog, and at some point I close the door in her face.

I'm sitting on my bed, shaking, not sure what to do. I'm afraid to go outside. I don't know if I should apologize. Yes, I've "disobeyed" her rules, but they are stupid rules, I'm an adult, and I don't think I've done anything wrong.

My phone pings with a text. It's from Linda. "Can you come out please? We need to talk."

Shit. The four worst words in the English language. I don't want to, but I can't hide in there forever. My heart is pounding, and I have a knot in my stomach from nerves, but I have to face the music.

I take a few deep, calming breaths and then I venture into the living room.

It's an unpleasant conversation. Linda tells me that she can't have someone living here who doesn't respect her boundaries. I tell her that I can't live here because it breaks my heart not being able to interact with a dog. We both agree that this isn't working and that I will move out by the end of the week.

I extract myself as soon as I can and go outside for a walk. I call Richard and start crying, relieved that I held it together until now. "I can't stay here this weekend," I sob, knowing full well that I don't have a choice. I'm on call

all weekend and can't leave. "Book a room for us at a hotel," he decides. "I'll bring the dogs."

I find a place that rents out little cabins by the river and is pet friendly. I rent one for two nights, pack my small suitcase and flee.

Having Richard and the dogs here is the medicine I need. We go for walks, have breakfast at an old-fashioned diner and dinner at a nice restaurant, and watch *Mad Men* reruns in between. I also obsessively check the Internet every few minutes for any new listings of places for rent. If I can't find anything I'll just have to live in a motel for a while. On Sunday night I say a tearful goodbye to them before going back to Linda's house. I could stay at the motel, but I already paid her the $500 and I have a feeling I won't be getting any of that money back (I'm right). Besides, if I don't return, she wins, and I can't let her win.

She's sitting in the living room, watching TV. I mutter a hello and go straight to my room. For the rest of my stay she acts as if nothing is wrong, trying to make conversation and even asking me if I want to eat dinner with her one night. I decline.

On Monday morning I tell my co-workers everything that happened over the weekend. They are satisfyingly outraged on my behalf, and what's even better, Emily has a solution.

"Charlotte is looking for a roommate," she informs me, referring to the woman who is working the other half of my rotation. I text her right away and we agree to a viewing the very same day.

The house is a rancher, located by the river, with a fenced yard. Charlotte has a dog too, but unlike Linda she has no problem if I want to play with him. Hurrah! We share the bathroom and living space, but the bedrooms are on opposite ends of the house for maximum privacy, and Charlotte tells me that she rarely stays there on her weeks off. But the best part is when she tells me that I can bring Lily, my corgi, with me. Even though the rent is a lot higher than what I had initially budgeted for, I'm so relieved that I've found such a good fit that I don't care.

A week later Lily and I move in. For the first time in thirteen years I'm living by myself again.

Sober Curious

Lily and I soon settle into a routine. She sleeps in her own bed next to mine, but every morning when I have coffee in bed she jumps up and snuggles close to me. We have a very enjoyable half hour together in which I sometimes journal or read, but most often scroll through Instagram. After that we go for a morning walk, usually along the river. It's very peaceful. Back at home I get ready for work, and then we drive the four minutes to the hospital. Lily stays in the car parked in the shade, ready for a lengthy morning nap. I walk her again during my lunch break and then after work.

This is the first job where I work alone, and I love it. I share an office with the lab staff so I'm not lonely, but I get to make all my own decisions and don't have to interact with anyone but my patients if I don't want to. It's absolute heaven for my introverted self, and especially needed after the socially overstimulated summer I've had at home. Most days I crash on my bed after work, reading and watching hours of *Grey's Anatomy*. I take lots of naps, sleep in on weekends, and live the sort of slow lifestyle I thought we would have after our move, but which hasn't really happened for us yet.

One Saturday morning I go to a coffee shop with my laptop to have breakfast and write. I've never done that before and want to indulge in this long-held fantasy.

The coffee shop is awesome: old wooden floors, mismatched wooden furniture, Tiffany lamps, and different merchandise lined up along the walls: pottery, funky jewellery, handmade soaps, local honey, and other cute knickknacks. The clientele is mixed as well: two bikers sit on the tiny porch, one digging into a huge plate of eggs, bacon, sausages, potatoes, and bread; the other delicately eating a bowl of fruit and yogurt. There is an elderly gentleman sitting in the sun, reading the newspaper, and sipping a cup of tea; a large group of tourists is noisily planning their day; a young family sits in a booth, the mother and daughter sporting matching boxer's braids; and another set of parents is playing a card game with their daughter.

I order French toast and a cappuccino, and then I sit down at a table by the window. It's ideal for people watching, which is what I'm doing for a while before opening my laptop and getting down to work.

An idea for a new book has cropped up, which is crazy. Didn't I just go through all sorts of anxiety surrounding the release of my first book? And yet here I am, ready to do it again. But I can't help it – I have the urge to write. It's something inside me that's beyond reason, something that's bigger than my fears and self-doubts. Elizabeth Gilbert describes that desire wonderfully in her masterpiece *Big Magic*:

"What do you love doing so much that the words failure and success essentially become irrelevant?"

For me that's writing. And for now I'm determined not to think about how and if to publish, just to get everything that's inside me and wants to come out onto paper. I never feel more alive than when I write down the chaotic thoughts in my head and transform them into words that make sense. There is no greater sense of accomplishment in the world for me.

My week in the little house by the river with my little dog has become my refuge. I'm only responsible for myself, my dog, and my job, which seems like an unbelievable luxury. From the time I was twenty-three I was caring for a husband, four stepchildren, a house, a farm, my husband's paperwork and working two jobs, then working while going to school, and then pursuing my career. No wonder I'm tired.

But being away isn't always wonderful: the weekends can seem endless, and I miss Richard and the rest of the dogs a lot.

Knowing I can't leave town due to having to be able to be at the hospital within 30 minutes in case of a callback makes me feel claustrophobic sometimes, like I'm in a cage I can't break out of.

I feel like my real life is put on hold half the time, which is good and bad:

I'm only available half the time for visits with friends, for being able to go somewhere, for looking after my own house and family.

And I'm not drinking seven days in a row, twice a month, which creates its own unique set of challenges.

* * *

My story with alcohol isn't one of great excess and even greater despair. It doesn't include arrests, DUIs, drunken one-night stands and a spectacular rock bottom. I suspect that my relationship with alcohol is one of millions. It's a relationship born of the normalization of alcohol and the omnipresence of it.

I grew up in Germany, the land of beer, wine, and Schnapps. My parents aren't big drinkers, and neither were their parents. I remember Mom and Dad sharing one bottle of beer for dinner during my childhood, and maybe adding a shot of rum to their evening tea if they were feeling wild. After my mom's diagnosis of rheumatoid arthritis she didn't drink for years, switching to non-alcoholic beer for their lone bottle of beer a night.

Alcohol held zero interest for me until I was well into my teens, when peer pressure and the desire to belong made me try some. I hated the taste but wanting to be part of a group is a powerful motivator, and I experimented with sweet liqueur, beer mixed with lemonade, and vodka in orange juice. I drank rarely and only when I was going out, which wasn't often.

By the time I was eighteen I had found my booze-legs. I had been adopted by the coolest group of girls in my high school, and they invited me to hang out with them almost every weekend. At the same time I also acquired a popular boyfriend who was part of a large group of guys who liked to party. Suddenly I was part of the it-gang, and I couldn't believe my luck.

We went out every Friday night, and my girlfriends had a ritual of pre-gaming before we hit the club. We spent hours in my friend's incredibly cool attic room, drinking cheap red wine, smoking cigarettes, gossiping, and laughing. We would paint our nails, do our make-up, put glitter in our hair and on our skin (it was the 90s), and talk about boys, school, and clothes. But most important of all – I was part of something. However, I never managed to become a full member of their clique, and I couldn't figure out why. I felt more like a beloved pet to them, someone they all liked but who was a step or two removed from them. Still, being invited was a thrill, and after a few glasses of wine I forgot that I was the odd one out. We would hug and sing and dance and declare our undying love for each other.

My popular boyfriend was sweet and loving. We stayed together for two and a half years, and I did most of my partying with him by my side. Alcohol became a big part of our nights out but was still limited to weekends only. It was further limited by my two weekend jobs: working at my parents' farmer's market on Saturdays meant getting up at 5 am and playing the church organ on Sundays meant getting up at 8 am. I was careful to not let my drinking get out of control because I knew I had to be fit the next day. And let me tell you, playing the church organ while hungover is its own special kind of hell. I did it once and never again.

During that time I had my first major depressive episode. I was going through an existential crisis, not knowing what I wanted to do with my life after school, and the shininess of the party life had worn off. The depression snuck up on me: things I used to love started losing their appeal. Going out? Don't feel like it. Hanging out with the guys at the skate park? What for?

I couldn't stand being with my own thoughts because they kept repeating how worthless, selfish, and useless I was. One time I went for a walk with our dog and the disc man I listened to ran out of batteries halfway through my walk. I panicked. I was so afraid of being the helpless captive of my vicious thoughts that I ran the whole way home. I have never been a runner and running up a long, steep hill made me feel like puking. But puking was about a million times better than having to listen to the voices in my head. I was seriously afraid of them.

Another thing that scared the hell out of me was when I couldn't focus on reading anymore. Books had always been my greatest love, and if they weren't there for me anymore, who or what was?

I didn't want to get out of bed, but my mom wasn't having it. "Are you sick?" she demanded, feeling my forehead. With no temperature and all my limbs intact there was no reason to stay in bed, and she made me get up. It cost me more energy than I thought I had. I started skipping school because I was sure my head would explode if I stayed in class and listened to the teacher droning on. I attached myself to the resident bad boy and we would drive to the lake, smoking and talking for hours, or go to the pub that was conveniently located three minutes away from school.

It never occurred to me that my regular alcohol consumption may have contributed to my depression, because I didn't know that I had depression. After a few truly horrendous weeks I slowly came back to life and promptly resolved to never think about that dark time again.

My alcohol consumption slowly increased during college, when going to the pub and to parties replaced going to the club. I started to enjoy the taste of white wine and tolerated the taste of beer, which was the cheapest drink.

When I met Richard I was catapulted from my college life to a grown-ass adult life. I learnt to cook, I looked after elementary school kids, I was suddenly a part-time mom and a full-time wife with a job and household to look after, and my drinking habits changed. Gone were the beer and the Jägermeister shots. We would have a civilized two drinks a few times a week, alternating it with nights of tea and ice cream. We went through a phase where we made our own wine and shared a bottle most nights. That went on for years. And then I crossed an invisible threshold that led to a subtle, but significant change.

* * *

I was in my early to mid-thirties now. I was in a great marriage, had a career I liked and hobbies I loved. There were also things that weren't great: I broke up with a toxic friend, which was the right decision but left me anxious; we had two teenagers and two young adults and the associated angst and challenges in our life; we were in a lot of debt; in the long months of the rainy and grey coastal winters I struggled with severe seasonal affective disorder; and there was the damn depression that would regularly visit me despite the antidepressants I faithfully took every day.

One Saturday afternoon I was alone at home, watching *What Not to Wear* with Stacy London and Clinton Kelly. They were chatting with their guest about how a particular outfit would be perfect for going out and having cocktails.

I could go for a cocktail I thought to myself, and then a rebellious idea popped into my head: why the hell not?

Up until that day I never drank alone. Alcohol was a social drink, only to be consumed in the presence of others. It was an unwritten rule in our family, one I had never questioned. But suddenly I was gripped by the tantalizing possibility of being reckless and a bit wild. Before I could change my mind I jumped up and raced to our wine cellar. Our "wine cellar" was the spidery bike shed attached to the house, a damp and dark place that was filled with lawn mowers, garden tools, old kid's toys, and other detritus such as tangled fishing rods, life vests and our old tent that had most of its parts missing. Richard had built a few sturdy shelves alongside one wall, and they were serving as our wine rack. We were into making our own wine at the time, and we had about 50 bottles of homemade red and white wine lined up on them. I grabbed a bottle of *Liebfraumilch* and sprinted back upstairs to make it back before the commercial break ended.

I pulled out the cork with a satisfying "plop", took one of our long-stemmed white wine glasses out of the cupboard and poured myself a glass. I put the bottle into the fridge and returned to the couch just as Stacy and Clinton came back with a new episode.

I took a sip and closed my eyes with pleasure. This was without a doubt the best sip of wine I'd ever tasted. Say what you want about our dusty and unstylish wine cellar, it kept the bottles nice and cool – the wine was the perfect temperature. But it was the thrill of the illicit, of doing something that I considered wrong that made the wine taste so good. Instead of being productive I was doing something decadent and self-indulgent, and it felt absolutely delicious. I put my feet up on the coffee table, took another mouthful and leaned back happily. This was the life! Nothing to do, nobody to look after, I didn't even have to get up early the next day. Just me, Stacy and Clinton and my friend Liebfraumilch, and not a care in the world.

But underneath the enjoyment, there was an undercurrent of trouble brewing. It was the faintest sense of threat, like a storm in the making on a clear day with not a cloud in the sky that only animals can sense. My sky was still blue, but something inside me could smell the danger lurking on the horizon.

All these years I could take alcohol or leave it, not being that terribly interested in it. I never craved it and couldn't imagine ever giving it greater importance in my life. By following my rule of only drinking with others there was always a certain amount of work involved: I either had to go out, which requires effort for an introvert and also included organizing a way to get home, or invite people over which meant cleaning the house, preparing food, and having to entertain. Staying in with tea and a good book often won out.

But now I had discovered a fateful new option: drinking alone. I didn't just like drinking by myself – I absolutely loved it. It felt like the biggest treat in the world with all my favourite things put together: solitude, watching something frivolous, getting the happy buzz of being tipsy, and munching on sweet popcorn.

When Richard came home two hours later he was surprised to find his wife exuberantly throwing her arms around him and kissing him passionately hello.

"Whoa, what's with you?" he asked in amusement.

"I'm just happy to see you!" I giggled and gave him another smooch.

He saw the almost-empty wine glass on the coffee table and comprehension dawned on his face. "Are you drinking?"

"Yes I am!" I said resolutely, ignoring the guilt I was feeling. "Want to join me?"

"Sure."

We ended the day sharing another bottle of wine together, having one of those beautifully animated conversations where you solve all the problems of the world and create magic together. I loved those conversations, and I was convinced that alcohol was *the* essential ingredient.

***

My relationship with alcohol changed after that experience. Once you have broken a rule, it will be easier to break it the next time. Before you know it, you have rewritten the rules so you can live your life without feeling guilty.

My wine consumption increased. I now thought nothing of it to come home and pour myself a drink, with or without Richard present. Justifying to drink by myself was easy since it's portrayed as completely normal wherever you look. Who hasn't seen any number of movies and TV shows where the heroine comes home, walks straight to the fridge, and pours herself a large glass of wine, to be consumed all by herself while looking thoughtfully into space? It's being hailed as the great stress reliever, as the special treat we all deserve, as #selfcare. Besides, "it's not drinking alone if the dog is home", and Lily is always by my side.

But I would be lying if I haven't secretly been worrying about just how much I look forward to wine at the end of the day, and I have noticed an alarming increase in my anxiety and worrying. I'm glad for the opportunity to take a break from drinking. Not only to give my liver a rest, but also to see how I feel when I'm not drinking a week at a time.

It's both easier and harder than I expected. Easier because there are great advantages to not drinking: I sleep better, I love waking up with a clear head, I'm much more creative when I'm not buzzed. My new book is coming along nicely, and I'm diving into a new genre of literature: quit lit, books about quitting alcohol.

I read *This Naked Mind* by Annie Grace first, which is taking a new approach to reducing alcohol in your life by debunking the myths surrounding alcohol and teaching the psychological and neurological impact it has. Annie promises that her book will give you freedom from alcohol by removing the psychological dependency, and I love it.

After *This Naked Mind* I read *The Sober Diaries* by Clare Pooley, a diary-style non-fiction account of Clare's first year of sobriety. It's funny and Clare's writing style is hilarious, and I enjoy it very much. I'm also intrigued by all the positive changes she's observed on herself: weight loss despite eating cake nightly, Hollywood-worthy shiny hair, and looking ten years younger – all by quitting her vino? Seems almost too good to be true.

Next comes *Girl Walks Out of a Bar*, the brilliant memoir of highly successful, heavily partying lawyer Lisa F. Smith. It's gritty and raw, honest and funny, and has some of the gnarly rock-bottom stuff of the movies: drinking first thing in the morning, doing plenty of cocaine, Lisa hightailing it to an obscure sushi place at lunch to down several jugs of sake to make it through the workday.

I read these books, do my journaling, go for walks, all the while wondering if this life – a life without alcohol – could be for me. But then the week is over, I drive home, and the first thing I do after kissing Richard and hugging the dogs is going to the fridge and pouring myself a glass of wine.

Because here is the hard part: during my week away I miss wine. My rotation starts and ends on a Thursday, and I'm always fine for the first couple of days. The weekend is usually okay too, but if I feel bored, I catch myself wishing for the easy distraction of a buzz. Monday arrives with the relief of a regular workday which means the day will pass by quicker than the interminable weekend I just endured. But then Tuesday arrives, and it's Black Day. It's hands down the most difficult day of the week for me. I've now been away from home for five days, and I'm done. I wanna go home. Everything sucks. I feel restless, annoyed, and frustrated. You know the feeling when you're stuck at the airport because your flight is delayed, and just when you think you can finally board, they announce that it's delayed by another five hours? And you are torn between exploding and bursting into tears? Yup, that's the feeling, *every second Tuesday*.

On those Tuesday evenings I'm convinced that quitting alcohol is stupid, that it would mean quitting all the joy and excitement in my life. All I can think about is all the fun times alcohol has given me: endless champagne during our last Mexico vacation. Cocktails with our friends on our Bahamas cruise. Ice-cold cider in my hammock on the sun-drenched porch on a hot summer day. Richard cheerfully calling to me when he's almost done with chores: "Pour us one, will you?" That delicious first sip when you come home after a tough day – or a good one, or a perfectly ordinary one.

Nights spent in front of the fire with Richard, putting the world to rights. Oh, fire drinking is one of my favourites, no matter if it's in front of the stove in the cabin or around a bonfire. Watching the flames flicker and dance is mesmerizing, only made better by the world dancing all around me with booze buzzing through my blood.

Is it any surprise that I go a little hard on my first day back? I deserve it after a week of abstinence. With the intoxication comes the 2 am wake-up with the self-loathing, and I did not miss that. Also, is it just my imagination, or is getting drunk not as fun as it used to be?

Because here's the thing: all the reading and reflecting and learning about the addictiveness of alcohol has made an impression. I'm not as ignorant as I was before, and now I have a little devil (or is it an angel?) on my shoulder every time I pour myself another glass, whispering into my ear that this is bad for me. Let me tell you, it takes a lot of the fun out of it. I manage to drown it out eventually, but just like clockwork the devil (it's definitely not an angel at night) will be there at two in the morning, a hundred times magnified, now *yelling* at me that I'M RUINING MY HEALTH AND MY LIFE!

* * *

That's my life for a year: a week of solitude, work, reflection, reading, writing, yoga, my fourteenth attempt at getting into meditation, naps, and Netflix. Followed by a week of being in ultra-social mood, hanging out with friends, drinking, talking nonsense, and doing basically none of the things that refuel me. While I do go for walks with the dogs, spend quality time with Richard, and enjoy being home, I barely do the little acts of self-care that have become part of my routine during my week away. It's not on purpose; I'm too busy and distracted to notice.

It's tricky to see the forest when you sit among the trees. But slowly I become aware of the stark difference between the two and start to wonder why I'm doing this.

Is it simply a habit? Have I fallen into the mindset of *I have to make the most of my limited time at home and I must have as much fun as possible?* That's part of it. As the months go by, I find the temporary separation harder and harder. I've committed to a year, and I'm determined to stick to my decision, but I often feel like my real life is put on hold half the time. I adopt an unhelpful "all or nothing" attitude when it comes to socialising, which is not me. As an introvert I need plenty of alone-time to recharge, but now I figure I can always recharge during my solo week.

The other reason is that I'm battling feelings of guilt for being away so much in the first place after Richard's illness less than a year ago. Am I a bad wife? Am I selfish? It makes sense financially and for my career in terms of my seniority, I know that he is okay with it, and I know that this is good for me, but I can't help it – the voices tell me I'm a bad person.

I'm relieved when my year away ends and determined to take the lessons I have learnt in my 194 days of clear-headedness and seclusion and apply them to my normal life. First and foremost on the agenda: to drink less. I've enjoyed the many benefits of not drinking, and I want to take that with me. To keep myself accountable I create a private blog I call *No more running with scissors* that I intend to use as a private journal of sorts. I'm excited, I'm motivated, I'm positive that I can do this – and I make a big mistake.

I don't tell anybody about my new resolve, mostly because saying you want to cut back/quit (I'm not yet clear on which one it's gonna be) implies you have a problem, and I can't do that. I have proven to myself that I can live and *thrive* without drinking – I've done that 27 weeks out of 52! So nope, I'm not addicted. I drink like most people, a lot less than some I know, and I'm not planning to cut back because I have to, but because I want to.

But another part of me doesn't say anything just in case I change my mind. Just in case I decide that my drinking is fine, and I've worked myself up over nothing, I want to keep the door open. I won't use it, obviously – but I want to have the option.

Reader, I will use the door again. Soon.

PMDD

I'm overjoyed at being home again. I love the freedom of no longer being tethered to the hospital 160 hours in a row without being able to leave town or have a bath in peace because I could be called in at any moment. I'm also overjoyed to have all the dogs and cats and Richard around me again every day. Lily is less impressed – she loved being an only child half the time and is not pleased that she has to share me again. My job status returns once again to casual with all the joys and uncertainties this entails. On paper it seems like a great option: you choose when you want to work, get all the time off you want, and don't have a set schedule. The flip side is that you have no guaranteed hours, and if you have anxiety that uncertainty is difficult to live with. I constantly worry about not getting enough work.

To ease my worrying I start to pick up shifts at a second hospital. It's another rural hospital in the village of Lytton, hundred kilometers away. I've missed the long drives through the beautiful landscape I love so much, which is like meditation to me. This new drive doesn't disappoint – I adore the winding road, encountering mountain sheep, half wild horses and one time a mama bear with her cub on my way to work. Bald eagles soar alongside my car above the river, enjoying their freedom, and I'm so happy driving next to them that I laugh out loud.

Lily is once again my faithful companion, lying contentedly curled up in the passenger seat or on my lap, happy to have my full attention which she is convinced is nothing less than she deserves. That dog can teach me a thing or two about confidence.

***

Lytton[3] is one of the oldest continuously inhabited areas in North America, with a First Nations history stretching back thousands of years. The Thompson and Fraser Rivers meet here which is considered the heart of the Nlaka'pamux territory. When the Gold Rush began in 1858, Lytton became an important spot for prospectors making their way north in hopes of finding a fortune.

It is now a sleepy town of 250 residents, but its history can be found everywhere. There's a small Chinese Museum that honors the significant Chinese presence that started with the building of the Canadian Pacific Railway in the early 1880s. The original hospital is one of the oldest in British Columbia, and the beautiful, ten-year old building that houses the hospital now has an interesting display of pictures, artifacts, and information about its history in the lobby.

The hospital is on the ground floor, and an apartment for staff is right above it. Two of the three doctors that rotate through come from out of town and stay in one of the three bedrooms, as do some of the nurses. I now join them several times a month. The apartment is cozy, with comfy couches and a TV in the living room, lots of squishy pillows and blankets to snuggle under, and a view onto the leafy courtyard. I spend many happy hours on those couches, Lily by my feet, because everybody who works there is a huge dog lover, and they welcome her with open arms.

During lunch and after work I go for walks with her through the pretty village. There's a tiny pink church, an eclectic gift shop that's so packed with merchandise that you have to squeeze through the aisles sideways, a diner, coffee shop, and a small supermarket. The historic hotel across the hospital has the best Chinese food, and just ten minutes away there's a baby waterfall I like to go to. Two railroad tracks go through town, and the frequent whistles

---

[3] Barbara Roden: A history of Lytton, from First Nations to the Gold Rush to disastrous fires, https://www.vernonmorningstar.com/news/a-history-of-lytton-from-first-nations-to-the-gold-rush-to-disastrous-fires/

of the trains coming through several times a day and night soon become background noise.

I like it there. I work alone again, with regular visits from Randy, the maintenance guy and Sybil, the lab lady. They're both locals and tell me town gossip and stories about the area and its people. I spent my lunch breaks in the shady courtyard, by the waterfall, or sitting by the river with Lily. If I stay the night we hang out in the apartment where I write, read, and watch TV. Spending only one night away as opposed to seven feels like a treat, not a chore, and everything is going well for a while.

Then I come home one day, see that the kitchen is a mess, and absolutely lose my shit. Richard isn't in the house, which is lucky for him, because I start yelling at thin air instead. The only witnesses are the poor cat and a couple of the dogs, and they all retreat at top speed. I'm incandescent with rage at the fact that *the useless idiot never cleans up after himself, why do I always have to do everything around here, I hate him, I hate my life, I hate fucking everything.*

I'm so furious I don't know what to do with myself. I'd love to channel Beth Dutton from *Yellowstone* and shoot the wind chimes, but we don't even have wind chimes.

I slam a couple of cupboard doors instead, but it's not very satisfying.

So I stalk to the fridge, pour myself a large glass of wine, down half of it in one gulp, refill it and then throw myself on the couch, glowering at the world. I silently dare my best intentions to say something about my behaviour, I fucking dare them. *Don't talk to me about mindfulness and feeling my feelings*, I growl at them, sipping aggressively. And they are wise enough not to.

I slowly, slowly calm down. I turn on the TV for background noise, scroll through Instagram and keep topping up my glass with the bottle that's now sitting on the table. No point in getting up every ten minutes for a refill – at the speed I'm drinking, the wine doesn't have a chance to get warm.

It takes me a while to realize where the rage is coming from, but eventually it dawns on me: it's my PMDD.

PMDD stands for **Premenstrual Dysphoric Disorder.** Dysphoria means being "in a state of unease or generalized dissatisfaction with life", and it sums up succinctly what PMDD feels like.

PMDD is a severe form of PMS, premenstrual syndrome. The difference between the two is that **PMDD is debilitating and severely affects the mental well-being** of women suffering from it. Up to 75% of women experience mild PMS, while less than 10% of women have symptoms that prevent them from functioning in normal life. (That number may be higher though; PMDD is notoriously under-diagnosed.)[4]

Just like Lyme disease a few chapters back, diagnosing PMDD isn't straightforward. There isn't a clinical test you can take that tells you yay or nay. Your doctor won't be able to do much for your diagnosis; you will have to do all the heavy lifting yourself. To figure out if you have PMDD you will have to go on a fact-finding mission that involves keeping track of your period, keeping a journal, and checking if your symptoms line up with the luteal phase. In case you're rusty on the different phases of your cycle here is a quick refresher: the average menstrual cycle is 28 days.

Days 1-7 are the menstruation, aka shark week in our house, which is part of the follicular phase (days 1-14). Day 14 is ovulation day, aka baby making day. The follicular phase is followed by the luteal phase, which is hell week when you have PMDD. Even though the luteal phase lasts two weeks, one tiny saving grace of PMDD is that it usually doesn't last the entire two weeks; for me it starts exactly one week before the onset of my next period on day 21, and as soon as that first drop of blood sees the light of day, my rage is over, at least for a little while. This part is important, because if your symptoms last into and past your period, you *don't* have PMDD. Lucky you! On the downside, you probably have a generalized depression/anxiety disorder. Life's a bitch.

Now that we've got the phases straight let's get to the fun part: **symptoms**.

The list of symptoms is long and varied, but if you have at least five of the following during the luteal phase, you have found your match made in hell[5]:

---

[4] WebMD, Do I have PMS, or is this PMDD?, https://www.webmd.com/women/pms/pms-vs-pmdd

[5] Johns Hopkins Medicine, Premenstrual Dysphoric Disorder, https://www.hopkinsmedicine.org/health/conditions-and- diseases/premenstrual-dysphoric-disorder-pmdd

- Depression
- Anger or irritability
- Trouble concentrating
- No interest in activities you usually enjoy
- Difficulty concentrating
- Moodiness
- Increased appetite
- Either insomnia or the urge to sleep all day
- Feeling overwhelmed or out of control
- Physical symptoms such as bloating, breast tenderness, or headache
- Feeling generally as if your life is suddenly three sizes too big for you and you can't handle it

I don't mean to brag, but I got all of them. It's ironic that the one area in my life where I'm an overachiever is something that affects my mental health and marriage in such a negative way.

Being diagnosed with PMDD is such a downer because it's a condition that doesn't have proper treatment even though it can be life-threatening. The cause is unknown as well, which is not helpful. The people who are in charge of discovering diseases think that it may be an abnormal reaction to the perfectly normal hormone changes that happen with each menstrual cycle. The increase in progesterone and estrogen levels may cause a serotonin deficiency – maybe? They're not sure. Cue shoulder shrugs all around.

The only cure is menopause, which means that there is at least one benefit to that beast. There are treatment options that can help relieve the severity of the symptoms, even though they won't be able to remove them completely:

- Eating a diet rich in protein and carbohydrates
- Decreasing sugar, salt, caffeine, and alcohol
- Regular exercise
- Avoiding stress
- Vitamin supplements such as B6, calcium, and magnesium
- Anti-inflammatory medicine

- Selective serotonin reuptake inhibitors (SSRI) aka antidepressants
- Birth control pill

I don't do nearly as well on this list as I do on the one of symptoms. Decreasing sugar, caffeine, and alcohol? Are they crazy? Chocolate and wine are what get me through every month without completely losing my mind.

Or are they?

Yes, my resolution to cut back drastically on my wine consumption was as short-lived as most new year's resolutions are. I went from a few days without, to just having a couple drinks, to right back to the old and trusted *go big or go home*. I'm home and I'm going big because there are just so many reasons to drink. I mean, did you not hear about the horror that I go through every month? A reason to drink if there ever was one.

PMDD and relationships don't mix well. I have friends who have PMDD, and they agree: nobody makes us as mad as our husbands do during hell week. I don't know if we subconsciously begrudge them their regulated hormones or if it's the whole Mars/Venus thing; all I know is that men can't do anything right when our hormones are in overdrive and that we are powerless against them. It's a lose/lose situation for everyone involved.

My friend and I both use a period-tracking app that gives daily updates on where our hormones are at. She texts updates/warnings to her husband; I tell mine in person (he doesn't do text) when the danger zone is coming. Forewarned is forearmed and knowing ahead of time that our hormones will be all over the place has made a huge positive difference. What's so terrible about the rage is that I always believe it. When it tells me that the world is a horrible place and my marriage is doomed, it feels like I see the truth for the first time. PMDD persuades me that I've lived a lie, and that what I'm experiencing now is reality.

* * *

Many years ago before we were married I actually left the house and stayed at a friend's place for a couple of nights during a particularly bad PMDD episode.

That was long before my diagnoses, when Richard and I didn't know what the hell was going on and didn't know each other very well yet. I believed the rage and left, thinking I would be better off without him. When my period came and with it reason, I went back with my tail between my legs. Neither of us had any idea what just happened – we felt like we'd just been through a war.

Not knowing what's going on with you is terrible. I have no doubt that undiagnosed PMDD has caused relationship breakups and destroyed careers. Spreading the word about it far and wide will not only save many women's (and their family's) sanity – it will also save lives. A global study published in BMC Psychiatry reports that 34% of women suffering from PMDD have attempted suicide.

Here is an excerpt from the UIC (University of Illinois at Chicago) article[6]:

"One of the big challenges with PMDD is that the medical community has not just been slow to understand this condition but even to believe it exists," said Eisenlohr-Moul, who is also chair of IAPMD's [the International Association for Premenstrual Disorders] clinical advisory board. "Providers and communities often dismiss patients' concerns, in part because women's complaints are less likely to be taken seriously than men's but also because of persistent and even sexist stigma and misconceptions around menstruation in general."

"PMDD is not a hormone imbalance. It is a neurobiological sensitivity to natural and normal changes in progesterone and estrogen levels," she said.

"Our study reveals just how destructive PMDD is," said Sandi MacDonald, co-founder and executive director of the International Association for Premenstrual Disorders. "This is a galvanizing movement in women's health. PMDD is a perfect storm where #MeToo and #TimesUp, meet mental health awareness, meets suicide prevention."

Premenstrual Dysphoric Disorder was finally included in the Diagnostic and Statistical Manual of Mental Disorders in 2013 as a major depressive

---

[6] UIC Today, Suicidal thoughts, behaviours linked to hormone-sensitive brain disorder, https://today.uic.edu/suicidal-thoughts-behaviors-linked- to-hormone-sensitive-brain-disorder/

disorder. However, as mentioned before, there are still way too many medical professionals who don't know (or don't care) that it even exists. Ignorance has always killed innocent people – and it's killing women who suffer from PMDD. There is no recommended standard screening of suicidal ideation in patients with the condition, and that needs to change.

I talk about it with women whenever I can. Almost none of them have heard of the condition, yet quite a few (definitely more than the "1 in 20" that's often quoted) think they have it. The average time for getting a diagnosis is 12 years – in my case it was 20, and only after my friend told me about it and I went to my doctor for confirmation.

There's a lot of work that needs to be done to spread awareness, understanding, and to stop with the misogynistic jokes about women and premenstrual symptoms.

"Women's troubles" have historically been disregarded as women just being "dramatic" or "delicate". But a few years ago a doctor (a male doctor no less) ruled menstrual pains *as bad as a heart attack*. Throw that into the next jerk's face who refers to women as the "weaker" sex: "Would you continue to go to work, raise kids and run a household while having a near-death experience and bleeding profusely *every month*? We've all seen you when you have a cold, Greg. So please STFU."

With PMDD you get the rage, depression, and suicidal ideation on top of the heart attack pain, and most women *still* show up to work.

We're the farthest thing from delicate or weak; **we are fucking superheroes.** But we could do with some help. This is a call for action to the medical community and society at large: please recognize PMDD as the debilitating, life-threatening condition it is. Please stop with the jokes. And please, for the love of God, find better treatment options. Until you do, women will continue to suffer and die.

Don't Should All Over Yourself

There's a saying in German: "When the donkey gets too comfortable he steps on the ice." It basically describes the human inclination to do something stupid when everything is going well, either out of boredom or because we aren't very smart as a species. I think about this saying often because it's just so damn true. Case in point: my latest decision. You would think that working in two hospitals, looking after a house, a farm, a husband, a recently injured dog, a new puppy, and my trifecta of mental health challenges would be enough.

But one day one of my co-workers bemoans the staffing shortage they have at the large hospital she's working at. She tells me about how stressed everybody is, how they are desperate for more people, and then she asks me: "Why don't you work there, Miriam? You would like it, everybody is so nice, and we could really use your help!"

Gosh, it feels nice being wanted, doesn't it? Someone asking me to be a part of something pushes all my *love me*-buttons, and without thinking much about it I agree. I apply and get hired on the spot.

This one is also one hundred kilometers away, and in case you are counting, this is the third hospital I'm working at that's within a radius of one hundred kilometers. There are a couple more, and at this rate I'll soon work at all of them. Why? I'm glad you asked, the reason is so compelling: because I think I should. I'm young(ish), I'm healthy(ish), I have no kids at home, I have time – why shouldn't I spend it on work, work, and more work? That's what I was taught growing up, and those lessons sunk in deep. Despite my best intentions I can never quite shake them off. Being at home more than two days a week when I could be working feels frivolous and lazy, and I'm still at the point in my life where I think those things are very bad.

What's ironic is that I just released my second book titled *Quit the Hustle*, which basically tells people to get off the hamster wheel and slow down. I mean it, too – but I seem to have some trouble applying what I'm preaching. Do as I say, not as I do, apparently. It's as if there's a disconnect between what I believe in and what I was brought up to believe – I'm still standing on the old side of the divide, trying to cross over but not quite making it.

When Richard was sick, I swore to myself that I would spend more time with him, because it was a painful reminder that our time together is limited. But then he got better, and I shoved that terrible period of our life into the remotest part of my brain, locked the cupboard and threw away the key. I couldn't deal with it, so I pretended it never happened. And with that avoidance technique comes the disregard of every good intention I had. I automatically resort back to what's deeply ingrained in me, and that is that I should work as much as possible, because being hard-working and busy all the time is the goal, isn't it?

There are good and bad things about this new job. The good ones are that I'm using the full scope of my skills again, which I haven't done in nearly three years. We are trained to work in the operating room, assisting the surgeons by taking live images of them fixing broken bones, putting pacemakers in, and operating on hearts, backs, and internal organs.

We also participate in special procedures like joint injections, studies of the digestive tract or taking pictures of the reproductive system. And we don't just x-ray people who are alive; we also occasionally x-ray dead bodies. Gunshot victims, people who have drowned or burnt, babies whose deaths are suspicious. Some days are heartbreaking and really tough.

Smaller sites don't do all of these procedures, but this big one does. It's challenging and a bit scary, but also satisfying as I get my confidence back.

But it's a lot. It's fall now, and the highway I take is the infamous Coquihalla highway, known as one of the worst roads in winter in all of North America. It gets extremely icy and snowy, the blowing snow eliminates visibility, and there are between 400 and 500 accidents every winter with plenty of fatalities.

You are required to have winter tires between October 1 to April 30, and with good reason: some of the worst accidents happen during spring break, when people from Vancouver wrongly assume that Easter means spring everywhere. I don't blame them: they've been living under blossoming cherry trees since February, and it's hard to imagine that the weather can be so completely different less than three hours away. But it is, and that mistake can be the last one they'll ever make. The Coquihalla is so notorious that it has been featured on the TV show *Highway Thru Hell*, and I've had plenty of its victims on my x-ray table with broken bones, head injuries or collapsed lungs.

One night I almost end up on the x-ray table myself. I work until midnight, and unbeknownst to me and my colleagues it has started snowing heavily. We work in a windowless department, so we are completely clueless to what goes on outside. A hurricane could tear through town, and we would be the last to know, only becoming aware once the casualties start to come in.

When the night technologist arrives she has snow in her hair and tells us about unplowed roads, vehicles in the ditch and a hill so frozen that cars are sliding down. I'm in trouble. The city is over 800 meters lower than the top of the Coquihalla, so if it's bad in town it must be atrocious on the top. It's midnight, I'm tired, it's snowing heavily, and the road conditions are terrible. I should take a hotel room for the night and drive home in the morning. That's what everybody urges me to do, and the left side of my brain agrees. But the same instinct that makes salmon swim against the current to spawn where they were born is telling me to go home, snowstorm be damned. "I will be fine," I say to my concerned co-workers, and *shut up* to my logical left side.

All I want is to sleep in my own bed. As long as I'm going slow I should be fine, right?

I've never been more wrong in my life. Just making it up the icy hill is a nail biter, and it gets worse from there.

The thing about the Coquihalla is that it is mostly pitch black. Contrary to what you may expect from a highway, it has no lights, no reflectors on the guardrails – hell, no guardrails for the most part. It's just a piece of pavement snaking across a mountain with some pretty steep slopes right next to the road, and if you're not careful you'll slide off and nobody is gonna find you in the dark.

I have an even bigger problem: I can't see the road. I'm in a blizzard, the first one of my life, and the timing couldn't be worse. I can barely see the road in my headlights, let alone anything else. I'm absolutely terrified. I put the hazards on and inch forward at a snail's pace, praying that the snow will stop. But that's still not the worst part. The worst part is when a vehicle is approaching from behind and passes me. The snow in its wake completely blinds me. Zero visibility, I can see literally nothing. I have no choice but to stop every time until the wildly whirling snow has settled, hoping that there isn't another car coming and hitting me. I'm a sitting duck, and I've never been so scared in my life. Tears are streaming down my face, and I keep muttering to myself *it's okay, you're okay, everything is gonna be okay*. I don't believe it.

It takes me hours to get home. Sometime around 2:30 in the morning I finally roll in, my entire body shaking and drenched in sweat. Richard is waiting up for me, clearly relieved to have me home safely. I break down in his arms. "I was so scared," I sob into his shoulder, and he rubs my back soothingly.

I stay in bed for most of the next day. I'm off work, which is lucky, because I wouldn't have been able to go in if I had a shift. While in bed I sip wine (for medicinal purposes) and ponder my options.

Is it worth risking my life driving on the most dangerous highway of North America because I think I should work as much as possible? Why do I even believe that I should do that? Who says? Why am I should-ing all over myself?

I have a running commentary in my head that never stops, like listening to a baseball game you can't turn off. My commentator is a woman, and alternately sounds like my mother, a mean girl, and a Stepford wife. They are always in there, yammering away, and what they're telling me is rarely anything helpful, let alone supportive.

Here's a little excerpt of a what it's like in my head right now:

Mother: *"Don't be so dramatic, it wasn't that bad. Hundreds of people drive this road every day, you're nothing special. Pull yourself together and get back to work."*

Mean girl: *"Look at you, lying around and feeling sorry for yourself. You're disgusting. And you're drinking in the middle of the afternoon like a common drunk. Are you an alcoholic? You are wasting your life."*

Stepford wife: *"What are you doing in bed? You're so lazy. Get up and clean the house, cook a nice meal for your husband and wash your hair. You're such a slob."*

They can go on for hours. The only way to shut them up is getting sloshed enough that I either can't hear them anymore or don't care. It's a flawed plan because of the inevitable comedown afterwards, but what in life is perfect?

* * *

I obviously go back to that hospital. Was there ever any doubt? Being a useful, hard-working member of society helps keep the voices in check, makes me feel respected by others, and is what I should be doing. Yup, I'm should-ing over myself again, I just can't help it.

When I'm doing too much, my body goes on strike by making me physically sick and forcing me to rest. I lose my voice for four days shortly after the blizzard debacle. A few weeks later my PMDD gives me horrendous cramps that keep me in bed for a couple of days. My depression contributes by making me not enjoy anything while I'm home: I'm restless, bored, miserable, and grey. Yes, grey is a mood that makes the world lose its colour, food lose its taste, and formerly beloved tasks lose its appeal. You are trapped in a cage of despair, and it takes all my strength to remind myself that this won't last. It always passes. All I have to do is hang on and wait it out – but it's hard.

Eventually the depressions fades away and colour returns. As my 40th birthday approaches I'm in a really good place: work is going well, I'm proud of myself for keeping all the balls (more or less) in the air and working my ass off; and it's Christmas season, which means guilt-free drinking. December is the month where anything goes, where cookies for breakfast and Baileys in your coffee are celebrated instead of frowned upon.

I ponder if I should celebrate my birthday by having a party, but ultimately decide that I'll keep it low-key and stay at home with cake, champagne, my husband, and my dogs. Hosting a party is giving me more anxiety these days than when I was younger, which is odd. I have way more experience in entertaining now, shouldn't it be easier? I also just don't have the energy. I've noticed that I seem to have less energy than I used to, but I blame it on work, turning 40, and life in general. The tiny voice in my head says that it's because of the wine and the associated poor sleep, but I dismiss that. I've never had a problem before, that can't be it. Maybe it's perimenopause?

* * *

For the new year, 2020, I make a few resolutions. I write a post on the blog where I share my "official" goals: writing a novel, moving my body regularly, getting plenty of sunshine and rest, doing yoga, wearing clothes that make me happy. All excellent goals, or more accurately guidelines I try to live my life by. And then there's a secret goal that I don't share: I want to drink less. Once again I don't tell anyone, not even Richard. I have no plan, I have no community, I have no specific why. Just a vague, nagging sense that I can't keep going on like this indefinitely. I'm hoping that I will wake up one day and simply don't feel like drinking for a few weeks, like it used to be. I used to go through phases where I went off booze for long stretches of time because *I simply didn't want to have a drink.* I would happily trade my wine glass for a bowl of ice cream or a cup of tea and not feel deprived in the slightest. Simpler times, am I right? I haven't felt like tea instead of wine for a WHILE. Isn't it about time that I'm hitting one of those phases again?

As it turns out, not this time. Without a plan, a reason, and a support system I last three days.

And then I say *Fuck it* and go right back to my old habits. January is hard enough as it is, no reason to make it any harder. What was I thinking?

Winter drags. January feels like the longest month in the history of Januarys, and none of them is short. Whoever coined the phrase "dog days of summer" had no idea what they were talking about. The days in January are the true dog days because every day feels like seven. I'm convinced I've aged a year, and at this rate I'll have reached menopause before the month is over. Richard will be a hundred years old. Clothes that were fashionable at the beginning of the month will be vintage by the end of it if the end ever comes. It sure doesn't feel like it.

Are we stuck in the hundred-year-winter of Narnia? Or in the movie *Groundhog Day*? Why does every day feel the same? I eat six square meals a day because every day is so long.

Is it any wonder I want to make the time pass quicker by drinking? Alcohol is a great antidote to boredom. The more you drink, the less you notice or care about the time. Hours suddenly fly by, and if you play your cards right you may even black out. Boom, a night gone just like that. I've had a few blackouts in my time, and generally don't recommend them. The panic of not remembering what happened, what you did, if you said or did anything embarrassing – it's very stressful. But in this never-ending month I can sort of see the appeal. Does January ever crawl in 2020 – snails move at lightning speed compared to it.

And wouldn't you know it, my depression is back. Sometimes I refer to my depression as my dark passenger. I'm a *Dexter* fan, and he calls his urge to kill his dark passenger. Mine doesn't make me want to kill, but it's just as relentless and impossible to escape.

Every New Year's I'm hopeful that *this* is the year where my

My depression always wins in the winter. No matter how hard I try, how determined I am, how much I count my blessings – it comes and claims me as its own. A weight settles over me. It makes moving hard. Getting out of bed difficult. Attempting new things nearly impossible. It dims the light. The world looks grey. People appear hostile.

dark passenger won't find me.

But every year I'm wrong.

I believe that everybody is out to get me. That everything I do will be wrong and just the excuse people have been waiting for to get rid of me. I'm scared of making mistakes at work because I believe that when I do everybody will at last realize what a failure I am.

I'm lonely.

At the same time, I also avoid people. As soon as I'm done with work I head home, eager to be alone. All I want is to hide from the world. I crave community but can't bring myself to go out and join other people. I try to remember that I'm loved, but it doesn't feel true. I'm suddenly convinced that it never was true, that everybody is talking about me behind my back, saying how annoying and selfish I am. That creates a

does its best to keep me isolated; it's much more powerful when I'm alone instead of having other people by my side.

I try to write but I have no energy, no creative spark, no concentration. I feel like a failure, a fraud, a silly idiot. My depression makes me feel like the biggest loser. I'm useless. I remind myself of my job, of my income. I'm productive, I'm a functioning member of society. I try to convince myself that I'm not useless. It helps a little, but not much.

My husband reminds me daily of how much he loves me. How important I am to him. It helps a little, but not enough.

My dark passenger brought his friend Anxiety along which means that my overthinking and worrying have gone into overdrive. I've read somewhere that worry is like praying for something you don't want to happen. Okay, got it, can you please tell me how to stop? Apparently not.

Anxiety makes me scared.

Scared of losing Richard. I'm always scared of losing him, but never more so than when I'm in the grip of my dark passenger and his friend.

I'm scared of not making enough money in the future.

I'm scared of getting sick.

I'm scared of my loved ones getting sick.

I'm scared of people confronting me.

I'm scared *all the fucking time.*

So I drink to forget. To drown out the voices of worry and self-loathing. To numb the fear that I feel all the time and that makes me crazy. There is no solution to a problem that hasn't happened yet. Nobody can guarantee me that nothing bad will happen to Richard or me, or our family, or our country, or the world we live in. In fact, bad things happen every day, and surely it's only a matter of time before we become one of the victims? Our luck is bound to run out eventually, right? When you really think about it, how can anybody remain calm and optimistic? Why isn't everybody screaming at the top of their lungs at the sheer magnitude of awfulness that's ALL AROUND US?

During the day I act my part: I smile, I'm friendly, I even crack jokes. I'm very good at hiding what's going on inside me. I might be a bit more quiet than usual, not as chatty; I'm probably complaining about being tired or stressed or feeling blah. I complain more about other people; I swear more. You can measure my declining mental state by the number of f-bombs I drop, but nobody knows that. Unless you live with me or know me well, I will look normal to you.

I'm like Dexter, my mask firmly in place. I blend in. Because my dark passenger is something that's not socially acceptable. Sure, we're now talking more about the importance of mental health. But it's something that's still more abstract than real. It's fine if I tell people about depressive episodes that happened in the past. They listen and nod and applaud me for being so honest. But what would they do if I told them that I'm having one right now? That I'm afraid I will yell at them to *shut up* because I don't think I can take them anymore? That it costs me everything I have to listen and nod and pretend that everything is normal? Would they still be understanding, or would I be hauled to HR before I can say *mental illness* and be disciplined for being disrespectful?

I have no idea. And I don't want to find out the hard way. So far I've managed to cling on by the skin of my teeth and never freaked out at work. I've cried, sure, but that's more easily acceptable. Especially when you tell them just one or two of the gazillion worries that have taken over your body and mind like body snatchers: that you're worried about your husband's health (always), a friend is sick (true), or you just can't stop thinking about whatever latest tragedy has everybody talking (wars, fires, floods, hurricanes, animals going extinct, people being murdered – take your pick). I obviously won't tell them that I'm feeling all of these at the same time, while simultaneously being in danger of losing my will to live. That would be TMI.

Dexter deals with his dark passenger by letting him take the wheel once in a while but staying right next to him, one hand on the steering wheel and one foot on the break. I'm dealing with mine by hiding in bed with a bottle of Sauvignon Blanc and something comforting to watch.

Neither system is perfect, but we make it work. Sort of. True, Dexter gets almost caught dozens of times and ends up dead, but it takes nine seasons before The End.

In my life I'm still only in season four, five tops – I have plenty of time before my dark passenger will catch me.

Right?

COVID-19

It's a Monday morning in March. The latest depressive episode has passed, which means my dark passenger and his buddy have retreated to wherever it is they're hiding when they aren't dominating my life. I'm working in the operating room at the big hospital that day.

Here's a little insight into what it's like working in the operating room as an x-ray technologist: it's uncomfortable. We x-ray techs are creatures of the dark. If you've ever had an x-ray you know that our rooms are dark, cold, slightly hostile caves. This is no accident; we like it that way. We as a species are loners who prefer to work in the shadows. There's no-one watching us when we do our job, just as it should be. The radiation keeps everyone away because most people are afraid of it. Is it swirling around in the air? Are we being irradiated all day long? How are we not freaked out? We give vague answers to these questions to keep the mystery alive (and also because we've forgotten the physics of it).

The operating room is the total opposite. It used to be called operating theatre (and still is in some parts of the world) because the early operating rooms were built gallery style for public observation. The horror! Even without the public watching, it's an environment as far removed from our dark caves as you can get. For starters it's so brightly lit, I want to get my sunglasses out. And there are so many people present! At minimum one surgeon (sometimes more), the anesthesiologist, a scrub nurse, and a circulating nurse. Quite often there are more nurses, a doctor assisting the surgeon, sometimes a sales rep who's peddling the latest in surgical equipment, and residents or students.

For some cases we set up in advance and take our images or videos unobtrusively while the surgery is in process, hidden behind our big machine and unrecognizable in our OR scrubs and masks. If everything is set up well we blend into the background, which is just the way we like it.

But then there are the other cases, the ones that give us nightmares. They are the ones where we have to come in mid-surgery and take x-rays that are essential for the surgery to continue. What this means is that everybody has stopped working and is waiting for us.

Imagine the scene: you get the call that OR 7 is ready for x-ray. You put on your mask, lead apron, and thyroid shield, grab the portable x-ray machine, and make your way to OR 7. Your heart is pounding, because you know in a moment you will be the centre of attention. You open the door, and there they are: half a dozen pairs of eyes on you. If you're lucky the atmosphere will be jovial, with everybody in there chatting and laughing, music playing, and a friendly hello directed at you. Those times are great.

But if the surgeon is in a bad mood you will be met with uncomfortable silence. Arms are crossed, which you know is to keep their hands sterile, but has a hostile effect, nonetheless. Maybe you will be greeted with an impatient "finally!" or "about time!" or "what took you so long?" You will apologize, even if you came as quickly as you could, and despite your resolve to stop apologizing so damn much. Sweat is starting to collect between your breasts and on your back. The lead apron is hot and heavy, but not as heavy as their merciless stare. If you were careless enough to wear your glasses today instead of contacts they will have fogged up so much that you can barely see.

You set up your equipment, which is never easy because the patient is nothing but a shapeless form under the sterile drapes. There's a light on the x-ray machine that outlines the area you will take the picture of. You turn it on but can barely see it because the OR lights are so bright, and your glasses are fogged up. You cross your fingers and hope for the best.

You walk around to the far side of the room, being extra careful not to touch anything and accidentally contaminating the sterile field. If they have to re-drape everything they will start throwing scalpels. On the far side you have to set up the imaging plate, again draped under a shapeless sterile drape.

You have to place it right next to the patient, usually in the spot the surgeon is standing in. You nervously ask them to move aside please. They glower but comply. You line it up with your machine on the other side of the patient six feet away, hoping desperately that everything is in the right place.

Everybody is still watching you. The lights are stupidly bright. You walk back to the front of the room, back against the wall, front to the sterile field. You double-check that you set the correct technique and then you take the picture. You walk back *again* to get the imaging plate, back to wall, front to sterile field. You leave the room with all eyes following you.

You are not done yet.

You jog to the machine that will read the information stored on the imaging plate and transform it into a picture. You stand in front of it and wait, heart racing, fingers crossed. If it didn't turn out you have to go back and repeat the entire procedure, which is humiliating. There is no worse walk of shame than that.

Phew, it worked! Sweet relief floods your system. You punch the air in victory before sending it to the computer located in OR 7.

You are still not done.

You speed walk back and enter the OR again. The six pairs of eyes lock on you questioningly. You nod modestly, but with triumph in your heart. Take that, suckers!

You walk to the computer where the surgeon is already standing impatiently. They can't pull the image up because they can't touch anything with sterile gloves, so you have to do it for them.

This should be simple, and it usually is, but there is one surgeon who wants everything displayed in a certain way which makes no sense to me. He sighs in exasperation as I fumble around, and I can tell that he's itching to just do it himself. You and me both, mister, but looks like neither of us gets what we want today. I finally manage, much to everybody's relief. He looks at all my hard work for ten seconds max before thanking me curtly. I'm dismissed.

I take the x-ray machine out of the room and slowly walk back to our work area. The adrenaline is rapidly draining from my body, leaving me weak-kneed. There will be several more cases throughout the day. Not all of them are that stressful, but the bright lights and audience remain. So does wearing the heavy lead apron, standing for hours at a time, and being at the beck and call of the surgeon. It's a far cry from our autonomous work environment in the x-ray department, which is why so few of us enjoy it. However, even fewer of us admit that we don't like going to the OR. It's a sign of weakness to admit it, so we all pretend that we are okay with it. "I don't mind the OR" is the most repeated refrain you will hear x-ray technologists say, but it is code for "I hate it, but I'll never admit it. Those surgeons don't scare me."

Back to that Monday in March. Despite everything I've just told you, I don't mind going to the OR. (And if I would I'd never tell you, so you will never know.)

The main reason is that one of my favourite co-workers is the permanent OR-technologist, and I love working with him. Jeff is chill and kind and patient, and we always end up having nice conversations in between cases. He's well respected amongst the OR-staff and being with him is like being with a B-list celebrity. (There is no other A-list except for surgeons in the OR-world.)

All humans likes familiarity, and surgeons are no exception. They know that he knows what they like, which makes everybody's life easier. I've been trained by Jeff, and because he's a good teacher – and I'm no dummy – I'm doing okay in there. Life is pretty sweet most days in OR-land, and today is a prime example.

We're hanging out in our tiny workspace, known as the alcove. It's minuscule, but that only adds to its charm. A small space fosters intimate conversations; it's a law of physics or something.

Jeff and I are talking about our weekend, and then he says: "Did you hear about the toilet paper wars?"

I shake my head and laugh. "The what? What are you talking about?"

"There's a video from Costco, I have to show you." He starts scrolling through his phone and then holds it out to me. "Here, take a look."

I take the phone and look in disbelief at the grainy footage. Middle-aged people are *racing each other* to the toilet paper display, throwing as many 30-packs as possible in their carts and hissing at anyone who comes too close.

There's a man trying to take a pack from someone else's cart, and they start fighting. A family has three carts piled high with nothing but toilet paper – they must have 800 rolls between them. What the hell?

I hand the phone back to Jeff. "What in the world is going on? Why is there a sudden obsession with toilet paper?"

"It's because of that new virus from China," he says.

"The coronavirus you mean?" I clarify. I've heard of a new virus that is making people in China extremely sick, but I haven't paid too much attention. I've had my own problems to deal with, and haven't there been other viruses in the past over there? They always go away after a while, don't they?

"The media is blowing this virus out of proportion, aren't they?" I ask Jeff.

He agrees. "I think so. People just have to use their common sense and wash their hands more often."

"And don't sneeze at each other, it's so gross," I add.

Then I return to the question that still puzzles me. "Why toilet paper? What does the coronavirus have to do with people in Canada going nuts about toilet paper?"

"I guess people are afraid that there will be disruptions in the supply chain, and we'll run out," Jeff shrugs.

We make a few more jokes about people clinging on to toilet paper like it's their firstborn, but then we're called in for the next case. As I'm getting suited up in my lead gear I can't help but mentally go over my own stash of toilet paper at home. How many rolls do we have left? Should I maybe buy some more just in case there will be a shortage?

Two days later, on March 11, 2020, the World Health Organization declares COVID-19 a worldwide pandemic. And the world as we know it ceases to exist.

At first it's eerily quiet in the hospitals. The hallways are deserted, the emergency waiting rooms are empty, our booking list has dwindled down to almost nothing. Talking to my friends at other hospitals I hear that it's like that everywhere; empty corridors, no wait times for the lab, more and more procedures being cancelled.

We are used to hustle and bustle, to every chair being occupied, to chattering and laughing and complaints about the long wait. We are used to running around and being busy.

The silence is unnerving.

We obsessively keep looking at footage from Italy, horrified at what we see. Field hospitals are being set up like in war zones. Patient stretchers line the hallways of overcrowded hospitals. Inflatable, sealed-off infectious disease tents are erected for the floods of critically ill patients.

Doctors are forced to make the devastating decision of whom to give a respirator to – leaving the ones without to die. There aren't enough beds in the intensive care units (ICUs), so the guidelines state that patients with the best hope to live should be prioritized.

We read about healthcare workers in China and Italy who have become infected and died. COVID doesn't seem to care if you are young and healthy – it can take your life anyway. And what about our middle-aged and older co-workers? What about staff that have asthma, or diabetes, or another pre-existing condition? Are we all risking our lives by doing our job?

Work emails and memos start flooding our inboxes daily with ever changing guidelines and new rules. Almost immediately there is a shortage of PPE, personal protective equipment. Instead of using single-use masks once (which is their intended purpose), we now use them for the entire shift, which means we have to keep them on even after having been exposed to contagious patients. Accidentally touching the front of the mask may mean getting infected. It's unnerving. There are little stations in our work area for every employee where we put our masks before going into the lunchroom, to be put back on after our break. We are told to wear eye protection or face shields, but there aren't enough. Many healthcare workers buy their own online. Some people bring safety goggles used for home projects and wear those.

There is a persistent rumour that we will run out of isolation gowns, supported by the sometimes-erratic new rules we're getting from management about when not to wear them. For example, if a patient comes in with COVID symptoms (we now call them "hot" patients) but doesn't cough, maybe we don't have to use a precious isolation gown?

The first time I have to x-ray a hot patient I'm terrified. I don't know yet if they have COVID or not, but we treat anybody with symptoms as if they do. It takes days to get the results of the COVID swab at that point, so we won't know for a while. I get dressed up in my mask, face shield, isolation gown (screw the guidelines about coughing, I'm *not* going in without a gown) and gloves, my heart pounding painfully in my chest. Am I about to face a deadly virus that could kill me?

The hospital has hastily been divided into hot and cold zones. Hot means infectious patients, cold means not. There is tape all over the floors and walls, and a new route we have to take if we're transporting hot patients.

I'm pushing the portable x-ray machine slowly along the red corridor, giving myself a pep talk. *You can do this; you're wearing your PPE; you will be fine.* I don't believe myself.

The patient is sitting upright on the stretcher in her cubicle in the ER. Her breathing is ragged; she clearly has difficulty taking a deep breath in. I want to turn and run away, but instead I greet her warmly and explain that I will be doing a chest x-ray right here in the ER, and that she won't have to do anything. I grab the imaging plate and approach the patient. She's wearing a mask; I'm wearing my PPE – but those thin pieces of cloth seem laughably inadequate protection against such a mighty enemy. Fortunately, now that I'm facing a patient who needs my service a switch has been flipped inside me. I can push the fear to the back of my mind and focus on the job at hand. I do the x-ray and leave with a mixture of pride and worry.

At home I've started stripping down to my underwear in front of the house, throwing the clothes straight into the washing machine and having a shower before saying hi to Richard or entering the rest of the house. For the first time in my career I bring my scrubs in a separate bag to work and get changed before and after work. Still, I feel dirty. Richard is 65 years old and has chronic Lyme disease. Could I kill my husband by bringing a deadly virus home from work? That thought keeps me up at night and gives me nightmares when I eventually fall into a restless sleep.

I seriously consider if I should take a leave of absence. But what if everybody would do that? Is that fair to my co-workers and patients?

I knew going into this job that I would have to deal with contagious diseases.

I've always been okay with that. But I didn't sign up to risk my life, or that of my loved ones.

Still, I keep going back, because really, what choice do I have?

We do the best we can and clean and disinfect all the time. Our hands are getting raw from washing them so vigorously and so often. I stop wearing my rings and put my wedding band on a chain around my neck instead.

And every time I'm on my way to work I'm queasy. What is waiting for me at the hospital? Is it starting to get bad?

Is today the day the wave will hit?

Cheers to the World Ending

Before the COVID wave hits there's another wave that's much more fun: a wave of love is flowing towards us!

Every evening at 7pm, people all over the world open their windows or step on their balconies to show their support for healthcare- and frontline workers. They whistle, bang pots together, and use cowbells or their hands to show their appreciation for everyone at the frontlines. It's very touching and makes us feel seen. Sure, sufficient PPE would be more helpful, but the pot banging is good for morale. So are the hearts appearing in windows everywhere, declaring people's gratitude. They are calling us heroes! We get free coffee, a discount on gas and first dips in the grocery stores.

The DIYers are having a shining moment using their skills to sew masks, hats, and uniform bags. A co-worker at the hospital brought in cute crotched headbands with buttons on the sides to attach our masks to that her mother-in-law made not only for her, but for us as well. Companies such as Apple, Dyson, and Ford are producing masks, face shields, hand sanitizers and ventilators.

After the first two weeks of a global lockdown, images are emerging of clear skies in India, jellyfish in the clean canals of Venice, Italy, deer walking past souvenir shops in Nara, Japan, and penguins waddling down the streets of Simon's Town, South Africa. Our battered planet is getting a much-needed break, and she clearly enjoys the respite from traffic and mass tourism.

There's solidarity everywhere. We are united against a virus that doesn't discriminate, and most people are doing their best by staying home, following the rules, and supporting each other as much as possible.

When I'm not working I thoroughly enjoy being home. After three busy years of frequent overnight guests and too much company for my introverted self I'm loving not having to entertain people. What a relief! I hadn't realized how much having visitors is work for me, no matter how much I like them: the cleaning and shopping and cooking before, during and after is not something I enjoy very much. I love our family and friends and like to see them, but getting this break right now is downright luxurious.

And you know what I don't miss? The dreaded unannounced visitor. It always irks me when people drop by without a warning. My house and I are *not* presentable every moment of every day. There is dog hair everywhere, but if I invited you I'll remove some of it before you arrive. I will also buy some good snacks and run a brush through my hair, and most importantly of all: I'll be mentally prepared to be social. If you just come without warning you will be covered in dog hair, get a stale cookie if you're lucky and be subjected to my sweatpants and monosyllabic answers. It's a lose/lose situation where none of us is having a good time. So yes, I'm loving the break from people spontaneously dropping by.

Plus, how cool is it to watch Netflix as much as you want *and* being considered a patriot for doing so? It's gotta be a first that lying on the couch and eating your weight in junk food is considered heroic.

And there's another thing: we are all drinking more. Opening a bottle of wine at lunchtime is all the rage now. We might die tomorrow, may as well go down having a good time, right?

Most people work from home now, having traded their business suits for yoga pants and their afternoon coffee for a cheeky glass of wine (poured into a coffee mug if you're on a Zoom call). With everything closed down we have to get our kicks somewhere, don't we?

A news anchor jokes that she ran out of toilet paper, but as long as she's not running out of wine all is well. Pandemic jokes about drinking are popping up like acne under our masks:

"It may take a village to raise a kid, but it takes a winery to homeschool one."

"Studies have shown that if you hold a drink in each hand you are 100% less likely to touch your face."

"COVID may be lung-related, but I'll sterilize my liver just in case."

"A bottle a day keeps the isolation boredom away."

Or the darker ones that contain an uncomfortable kernel of truth: "You can't die of COVID-19 if you die of alcohol poisoning first."

All the jokes and references to our increased alcohol use seem funny, but they are highly problematic. It normalizes drinking even more than it already is, and it gives us the perfect excuse to throw caution to the wind and go nuts. Everyone is doing it, why not me?

The truth is that we are all freaked out. The lockdown keeps getting extended, the amount of people infected and dying keeps rising, and people are starting to go stir-crazy being stuck at home. Time passes, and instead of things getting better they keep getting worse. Easter is cancelled, and everyone is willing to sacrifice that holiday. But now we are faced with the possibility that we may not see our families at Christmas, which is still months away, and the realization that this pandemic is not going to be resolved as quickly as we initially hoped is depressing.

And what's the quickest way to cheer yourself up? Pour a drink, of course. It gives us temporary relief from the depressing news, and after a few drinks we stop caring so much.

We don't want to deal with the reality that the world as we've known it is irrevocably gone. We'll never return to the way it was. We are disillusioned and disappointed, and we need an escape.

Booze gives us that for the first little while, but once that's not enough anymore we are looking for a scapegoat. Enter: conspiracy theories.

The solidarity I mentioned a couple of pages ago is short-lived, and barely a month into the pandemic conspiracy theories abound. COVID is fake, or it's engineered by the Chinese for world domination; it's spread by 5G networks or created by big pharma for big profits. My favourites are the videos that are "only streamed for 24 hours before the government will shut them down". Totally normal, right? Aren't all authentic news taken down after 24 hours?

In a way I get it. I understand the desperate search for answers that may lead you down some questionable allies. We want someone to tell us what's what, and most importantly, *when it will all end*. The not-knowing is playing tricks on all of us. And it wears us out.

We're exhausted.

Being scared all the time is exhausting.

Disinfecting, cleaning, washing hands, worrying about what you have touched – *did I sanitize after leaving the store? Did I wipe down all the groceries before putting them away?* – is exhausting.

Worrying about getting sick and accidentally killing your husband is exhausting.

Working while wearing a mask, goggles, gloves, and a gown is exhausting.

Stripping down on your doorstep, throwing your clothes in the washer, and having a shower before you can even hug your family is exhausting.

And the sheer number of patients we are getting again is exhausting. Yes, the patients have returned with a vengeance, and they brought their friends. The emergency waiting rooms are full to capacity again, all the hospital beds are occupied, and the ICUs are over capacity. Just because COVID is running the show doesn't mean that all the other diseases are on vacation. Cancer, heart attacks, strokes, accidents, and hundreds of other illnesses are still around, and patients still need to be treated for them.

Many people had their elective surgeries cancelled due to the pandemic, and they are understandably frustrated. Unfortunately, some of them choose to vent their frustrations on us, which is not only useless (I'm an x-ray technologist with zero power) but also draining our already depleted energy reserves. Trust me Karen, I know how you feel, but there's nothing I can do.

Other people are nervous about being at the hospital and getting infected, which is also understandable. They require extra attention and reassurance, but how can you pour from an empty cup? Our cups are empty, yet we are still dealing with thirsty people day in and day out. Somehow we find some more in us to give, but now we are running on a deficit. How long can that last? How long will we?

We still have hot and cold sections in the hospital, and every single person that comes in with any possible COVID symptoms – cough, fever, loss of smell or taste, difficulty breathing – has to be treated as a hot patient, which generates a lot of extra work. They have to be isolated, every person that comes in contact with them has to put on PPE, the patient can't leave their isolation room and no family can come in. A commode has to be brought in when they need to use the bathroom because we can't let them use the shared bathroom. Once they are discharged the rooms have to get a deep-clean, which takes time and extra cleaning personnel. It's draining. The good news is that we finally have sufficient PPE – the bad news is that we go through it rapidly.

By the time I get home after a two-hundred-kilometer round trip and an eight-hour shift, a shower and laundry, I have no energy for yoga or a walk or meditation. So I do what everybody else seems to be doing in this pandemic: I pour myself a large glass of wine and try to drown my sorrows.

I've switched to boxed wine because it's more economical, and the bottles were getting out of hand. Also, I can lie to myself better about how much I'm drinking because it's harder to tell. At first, a four-litre box of wine (equivalent to five-and-a-quarter bottles) lasts a week. Well, sort of. If I buy a box on Monday I usually buy another one for the weekend, especially if I'm off work. Just in case guests come over, you know? We have a few people in our bubble who we are hanging out with again, and they are wine drinkers as well.

But even without anyone coming over, the box seems to empty at an alarming rate. Is there a hole in the bottom? I shove that worry deep down where everything else goes I don't want to deal with. They call that place the pit of your stomach, which seems fitting; a pit is a hole where dark and dangerous things happen (think bear pit, pits where animals are forced to fight, a barbecue pit filled with burning wood and hot coals). I have no idea how deep my pit is, but I hope it's nice and roomy. I have the distinct feeling that plenty more stuff is coming that I need to store in there.

I justify my increased wine consumption by reminding myself that we are in a pandemic, that I'm *risking my life every day* (and that of my husband, but let's shove that fear down into the pit), and that everybody is doing it. Yes Mom, if everybody jumps off a cliff I would follow them. Who wants to be left behind?

There's another reason why I'm drinking more.

On paper it looks like I have everything. I'm happily married, we are debt-free, we are reasonably healthy, and I have a good, safe job. Well, safe as in that it's recession-proof; it has the downside of possibly infecting me with a deadly disease. Nothing is perfect, am I right?

My job as an x-ray technologist is important to me. It's not only what I do but also part of my identity, my income, and maybe most importantly, my source of self-worth. I'm proud to be an x-ray technologist, especially in these challenging times. I'm also proud to be the one bringing home the bacon since Richard's retirement. I always assumed that I would play second fiddle to my husband's income. That he would bring home the real money, while I would bring in substantially less. His Lyme disease diagnosis changed that. While I always knew that he would retire decades before me, we thought he would work several more years. But we make plans, God laughs, and now I'm the main bread winner.

The responsibility weighs heavily on my shoulders. The fear of unemployment, financial ruin, and the collapse of society as we know it is always at the back of my mind. So I try to prepare as best as I can by working lots, making as much money as possible, and burying all the nuts I can like a squirrel, until the arrival of the inevitable catastrophe that's surely waiting just around the corner.

What that leads to is that I'm neglecting an important part of myself. I need to write to make sense of myself and my confusing thoughts, to find out what I'm thinking and what it all means. When I'm not giving myself the time and space to do that I'm floundering. I get lost in my own head, drowning in my thoughts. You've gotten a little glimpse into my mind, and how my mental illness manipulates my thinking, and it's no fun in there if I don't get the chance to clear it out by writing everything down. Writing is like Marie Kondo-ing my head. I take everything that's in there, lay it out in front of me, and then go through it one by one. If it doesn't give me joy, it's gone.

Ha, I wish! If it would be that easy I'd have no problems. Still, while I can't just give away my anxiety, overthinking, self-worth issues and fear, writing helps me to put things into perspective. It shows me what's real and what's imagined, what is a problem that needs to – and can – be dealt with, and what is something that exists only in my head.

But I haven't been writing because I've chosen work. And the reason isn't only money and the need for healthcare workers, it's also something else: I've chickened out. I don't know if it's worthwhile to continue with this writing thing. Despite having written two books, dozens of articles, and thousands of blog posts I still feel like an amateur who's playing around. That may be acceptable behaviour in normal times, but during a pandemic it's downright frivolous to indulge in such an unlikely dream. Writing is nothing more than a little hobby, and hobbies have to take a backseat to real life, right? It's called being a responsible adult, and it's about time I stop dreaming. Having your head in the clouds doesn't pay the bills but accepting another shift instead of staying home and "trying to write" does.

Besides, who cares in these times if I write or not? Writing doesn't matter. My earning potential and service to society do.

By working the socially accepted job with the set wage, I get social validation. This is a path my parents understand. Writing about myself? They most definitely do not understand that.

I am known as a good, reliable employee. The public calls me a hero. (That's starting to change, but more on that later.)

I'm fulfilling my responsibility as a mature, considerate citizen of my country by doing my part.

But it's breaking my heart. I desperately miss being creative. It's a part of me that elevates my life from just existing to really *living*. Sure, my basic needs are being taken care of, I have food, water, shelter, clothing, employment, family support and social stability. I have love and friendship. I know how lucky I am, and it feels greedy to want more.

But I do want more. And it feels more like a need than a want. It feels necessary.

I don't realize it at the time, but art is much more than an extravagance. What are we doing during lockdown? Watching movies and TV shows. Listening to music and podcasts. Reading books. Italians are singing together from their balconies and windows to feel united and boost morale.

All of this is art. Painting, sewing, baking, doing arts and crafts is what helps us find joy amidst fear, uncertainty, and boredom.

Me choosing work over writing is not doing me or anyone around me any favours. I'm denying myself one of the most important morale boosters I have in my mental toolbox. It's what would refill my rapidly depleting energy reserves, and by denying myself that I'm actually decreasing my usefulness as healthcare worker, wife, and human being. You can't pour from an empty cup, and I'm not doing the thing that helps me refill my cup.

As a result I'm getting depressed, and I self-medicate to numb the depression. The alcohol makes the depression worse, which in turn leads to more self-medication. It's a vicious cycle I can't seem to find my way out of. As much as I hate to admit it, I need help.

It's time to face another one of my fears: therapy.

Gifts

How do you start therapy? I have no idea. When I asked my doctor the previous year about therapy he mentioned a practice in town, but I'm reluctant to go there. I live in a small town, and the chances of running into people you know are high. What if I see my therapist in the grocery store? What's the protocol? Do I ignore them? Make small talk? I don't like small talk at the best of times, I can't even imagine how excruciating it would be with someone who knows my darkest secrets. No thanks.

I google "therapy", and 805 *million* search results pop up in 0.69 seconds. Huh, at least I'm in good company. But having too many choices is almost as bad as having none because they paralyze you. The thing about being in a depression is that you are unable to make simple decisions such as if you should have a shower or not, so making an important one like whom to confide your messed-up mind to is impossible. How would you ever find the right one?

Unhelpfully, my mind immediately starts conjuring up worst case scenarios: a therapist who laughs about my insignificant problems, telling me to stop wasting their time. Or it might be a therapist who confirms my biggest fear, that I'm a horrible and selfish person. A therapist who hypnotizes me into doing things I don't want to do. (I saw that in a movie once; the therapist in question made his patients commit suicide. It was horrible.)

I'm thinking of every movie I've ever seen with the quintessential genius therapist with a bushy beard, tweed jacket with elbow patches and an absentminded manner. Their offices are either messy (to symbolize their ineptitude of mastering daily life while underlining their genius status) or stuffy, dark wood panelled affairs, and they always have an uncomfortable looking couch for the patient to lie down on.

Their method is to sit there in silence with pen poised over notebook, and when the patient tells them something, *anything*, to ask "how does that make you feel?"

There's a loudly ticking clock on the wall for the patient to stare at while the bearded therapist is staring either at the patient or out the window. It's my version of hell.

If it's a female therapist they're either old, resembling a stern head mistress, or attractive businesswomen with sharply tailored suits and high heels, impeccable make-up, and a thinly veiled impatient manner. They had to work twice as hard for half the recognition than their male counterparts, and they're still angry about that. You are nothing but another opportunity to prove their competency. You better heal and be one of their success stories or stop wasting their time.

Then there's the hapless hippie-ish therapist with long hair who wears long flowy skirts, clogs, and oversized cardigans. She is an idealist who cares deeply for every single one of her patients which often gets her into trouble by being too involved. She will have fresh flowers and homemade, slightly burnt cookies in her office, instead of a couch you sit in an IKEA Poäng armchair, and she will look you in the eye and earnestly promise not to rest until she has helped you.

None of these versions are inviting. I close my computer, defeated. Maybe I should just increase my dose of antidepressants as recommended by my doctor and hope for the best.

But once I have an idea it stays with me. No matter how much I try to ignore it, it niggles away at me in big and tiny ways. It's that way with a book that wants to be written by me and will continue to knock on my door like the most persistent Jehovah's Witness determined to save me. The idea is like a physical presence inside my body. I can feel it in my belly, my brain, and my fingertips. My belly will flutter like there are a million butterflies in it, or contract painfully when I don't respond, or curl itself into a ball of anxiety in the pit of my stomach. It's impossible to ignore.

My brain will send me messages in my dreams every night, showing me what I should do, and nightmares showing me what will happen if I don't. I will go into trancelike daydreams when I'm walking or driving or tipsy. Those dreams show me what could happen if I take the idea and run with it.

I'm restless and unable to fully focus on anything but the idea. It's always there: while I'm at work, doing the dishes, trying to read a book. I spend countless hours thinking about it and resisting thinking about it, and at some point I realize that I could be done by now if I'd used the time I agonized about the idea and just did it already.

My fingertips itch with eagerness to get started. They are sending messages to my brain to elicit its help. *We are ready*, they tell Brain. *Make her use us already!* Brain keeps sending me dreams and nightmares and daydreams and conspires with Belly to keep twisting and fluttering and knotting.

That certainty I get to follow an idea is a gift. It's bigger than me and my logical brain, bigger than my fears and imposter syndrome, bigger than my environment and the limiting beliefs I was taught. It's one of the jewels buried inside me, and I believe it's the other side of the coin that is my mental illness. Everything has two sides, and I choose to believe that my mental illness has come bearing gifts, not just hardship.

Being open to receiving an idea when it knocks on my door is one of the gifts it has given me.

I'm tuned in to my inner body despite doing my best to numb it with wine, and it feels nothing short of magical.

The sensitivity I have to life's tribulations comes with an upside as well: I'm just as receptive to life's triumphs. I experience pure joy when I see the sparkle of a million snow crystals in the sunshine, when I drive past a herd of half-wild horses with their foals, when I feel the warmth of the spring sun on my bare skin.

And then there is the gift of being able to express on paper what is on my mind.

Writing is a sacred, enchanting process to me: more often than I can count I've sat down to write about one thing, and something entirely unexpected has flown out of my fingertips.

I've always loved this Joan Didion quote:

"*I write entirely to find out what I'm thinking, what I'm looking at, what I see and what it means. What I want and what I fear.*"

She put it absolutely perfectly. That's exactly what writing is for me, too.

And now my gift is that the idea of therapy won't leave me alone. Something wise inside me knows that it will help me. Tara Mohr calls that wise voice our *Inner Mentor* who unfailingly provides us with ALL the answers to our biggest challenges.

My Inner Mentor is gently urging me to get my head out of my ass, stop with the pessimism and just *do* it. Who am I to argue with my inner wise woman?

Since I still don't know how to find a therapist I ask the Internet for help. I put the question on my Instagram stories if anyone has recommendations for a therapist, and my friends deliver. Two share their therapists with me, and I pick the one who is older, rationalizing that older equals more life experience. I'm incredibly nervous as I send her an email, asking for help to deal with my anxiety and depression. Tori replies within hours, and we agree on an appointment the very next week. Fortunately it will be on Zoom (thanks COVID!) so I will avoid the dreaded couch. I figure that if it gets to be too much I can simply shut my laptop and never contact her again.

It's unbelievable, but true: I'm going to have my very first therapy session in a week.

I'm terrified.

Therapy I

My biggest worry is awkward silence. What if she just stares at me through the screen and I don't know what to say? Will she have a large clock in the frame for me to watch the minutes tick by in agonizing slowness?

The day of the session arrives way too quickly. I position myself on my living room couch (the irony) with a glass of water and tissues. I figure I'll need them, and I'm not wrong.

I click on the link she sent me via email, and the minutes before she lets me in the meeting are pure agony. I'm so scared I'm afraid I might have an accident. Let me tell ya, being scared shitless isn't just an expression. I wonder if I have time to go to the bathroom, but what if she appears and I'm not there? I figure I better hold it.

When I'm nervous I get shaky, my stomach hurts and I regret every decision I've ever made that led me to this point in time. Now I'm cursing my Inner Mentor for making me do this. What a bitch! I'm trying some deep yogic breathing to calm down, but it's no use. Maybe I should have had a shot of Tequila for courage, isn't that what Jennifer Lawrence did before she won her Oscar? But then she tripped and fell on the stairs, so maybe that's not such a great idea.

While I'm contemplating to slam my computer shut and run, the screen suddenly comes to life – and there she is. Tori is a blond, pretty woman in her forties, and she greets me warmly with a big smile. To my horror, I burst into tears before I can even say hello.

"I-I'm s-s-s-o s-s-o s-s-sorry," I hiccup, trying desperately to stop the tears, but it only gets worse. I'm cringing with embarrassment, but Tori is unfazed.

"I'm very comfortable with tears," she assures me, and hearing that does make me feel a bit calmer. Instead of watching me silently as I've been afraid of, she chitchats cheerily, telling me a bit about herself, her office, and commenting on the weather. She asks me if the lighting is okay, and as I answer in the affirmative I notice to my surprise that I've stopped blubbering. She's good!

"So, what's been going on?" she asks eventually. "You mentioned anxiety and depression in your email, and I can see that you are in crisis. Tell me about it."

I don't know where to start. I haven't really thought through what I want to say, because I don't know what's wrong with me. So I start with my depression diagnosis from eight years ago. I tell her how high-functioning I am (I can't help myself; this is so important to me), but that working as a healthcare worker during COVID is harder than anything I've faced in my career thus far. She nods encouragingly and says that many of her clients are fellow healthcare workers – she gets it. I mention the increase in depressive episodes and my worry that my antidepressants aren't working anymore.

What I don't mention is the increase in my alcohol consumption, but I keep expecting her to ask me about it. It's at the forefront of my mind, and it feels as if it's written on my forehead. *Don't you want to know how I deal with my stress?* I keep thinking, equally terrified of the question and anticipating it. As I'm recounting some of my stuff, I realize for the first time that this is the main reason I've contacted her – I'm worried about my drinking, and I need to confess my worries to someone. Richard doesn't know the extent of my secret drinking, and when I've asked him if he thinks our boozing is okay he always says it is, and that I worry too much. I'm way too conflicted about it to confide in anyone else, and as I'm sitting here, babbling away, it's dawning on me that I'm not ready to talk about it to her either. If she doesn't ask I won't tell, and I'm suddenly panic-stricken that she might mention it. *I don't wanna talk about it!* I telegraph to her, and she must have received my message, because she never asks anything about drugs or alcohol.

As it turns out, there is plenty to learn about anxiety and depression without getting into the gnarly subject of self-medication.

Tori is teaching me about thoughts. She says that we have thousands of thoughts every day (tell me about it, sister), and that we drop the vast majority of them, never to be thought of again. For example, I may get briefly annoyed at the driver who passes me even though I'm already over the speed limit, causing me to give him the finger (but below the steering wheel so they don't see it – passive-aggressiveness or self-preservation? You decide).

But a minute later I'll have dropped that thought and it's gone.

If we hold on to thoughts we turn them into beliefs. Tori explains that beliefs box us in. They are limiting. Beliefs leave no room for other interpretation because *we already think we know the truth.* For example, if we believe that anything worth achieving requires a lot of hard work and sacrifice, we won't even question that thought. To us it's a fact of life.

Tori picks up a pen from her desk and holds it in her outstretched fist. Then she opens her fist and lets the pen drop onto the desk. "See?" she says. "It can be just as easy to drop a thought or belief as it is to drop this pen."

According to her we choose which thoughts we hold on to, which sounds great but is also a lot of pressure. Are you telling me I'm *choosing* to be miserable?

Tori says I have the option to let go of *any* thought whenever I want to. She tells me about clients who have been able to release severe traumas such as rape or abuse, trauma that in some instances happened many years ago and significantly overshadowed their lives until they made the conscious decision to release it. Years and years of trauma gone in an instant – poof! Just like magic. I must look skeptical, because Tori laughs and promises to share this miracle cure with me right this minute.

"Have you heard of *The Sedona Method*?" she asks.

I shake my head no.

The Sedona Method is the technique to get rid of whatever it is you don't want anymore, like a powerful all-in-one cleaner. Doubts, unwelcome thoughts, old beliefs – you don't like it, drop it like it's hot! It promises to unlock joy and happiness and get rid of all the nasty stuff you have no use for.

How? By answering three questions:

1. Could I let it go?
2. Would I let it go?
3. When?

I wait for more, but that's it; just these three very simple questions. I'm unconvinced that this works, which is handy, because I can use the Sedona Method to let go of that doubt once and for all.

Let's try:

Could I let go of my doubt? I ask myself: Does the doubt serve me in any way? No. Would it harm me if I'd let it go? No. We have established that nothing bad happens if I let go of that doubt, so the answer is yes, I *could* let it go.

Second question: Would I let it go? That's the tricky part where I'm getting defensive. Tori says it's up to me to release it – I say it's not that easy. Where's the switch I can flip, or the trapdoor I can open through which all my problems just whoosh out, never to be seen again? I can't find them. She looks at me expectantly, waiting for my answer.

"Well, of course I *want* to let go of it," I squirm. "I just don't know how."

Tori picks up her pen again and demonstrates letting go by dropping it on the desk. "Just like that," she says unhelpfully. I hide a scowl with difficulty. I'm not sure I like therapy.

I never get the hang of the Sedona Method, but Tori helps me in other ways. We go back to my childhood (you really do that in therapy, I had wondered) and uncover a few important facts that explain a lot. I was a sensitive, fearful child, and instead of taking me the way I was, my parents tried to "toughen me up". My mom didn't believe in indulging my many fears and got impatient at my terror of social interaction. My parents own and operate a grocery store and having to go in and interacting with customers was torture for me. I was happiest curled up with a book far away from other people, but that wouldn't do. I had to be there every day after school and starting at age twelve I had to work at the Farmers Market every Saturday, selling produce. I woke up with stomach cramps every Saturday for years because I was dreading it so much. It was a busy market, with customers clamouring for attention, and to me it felt like being thrown into a pit of wild beasts.

You had to ask loudly who was next in line, which was pretty much impossible for me. I couldn't find my voice and stood frozen to the spot until Grace, a kind, cheerful woman who worked for us for decades, pointed me gently to a customer who needed help. Without Grace I would probably still stand in that same spot, eternally frozen, a warning to all the other sensitive girls who couldn't make it in this world.

I eventually found my voice, and in my later years learnt to actually enjoy the work. I liked the camaraderie, the fast pace, and the money – my dad paid well. I've always believed that without being pushed to do that I would have turned out to be a very different, much more fearful and, if that's possible, even more insecure woman.

But it came at a heavy cost. If your feelings are regularly invalidated, you learn not to trust yourself, which is dangerous. If you don't trust your own instincts and believe that your feelings are wrong you look for guidance outside yourself. That makes you easy prey for controlling men, selfish friends, and gaslighting. If a friendship is one-sided where you always give and the other person always takes, you might not trust yourself that you're seeing the situation correctly. Especially if the friend turns it around and accuses *you* of being the user, you might believe them because you were taught not to trust yourself.

I've been on the receiving end of gaslighting several times before I even knew what gaslighting was, and it's only in recent years that I'm starting to recognize it and trust myself more than other people.

What *is* gaslighting? The American Psychological Association (APA)[7] defines it as follows:

"To manipulate another person into doubting his or her perceptions, experiences, or understanding of events. The term once referred to manipulation so extreme

---

[7] APA Dictionary of Psychology, https://dictionary.apa.org/gaslight

as to induce mental illness or to justify commitment of the gaslighted person to a psychiatric institution but is now used more generally."

It's an insidious way of sneakily misleading a person into questioning their judgment and reality.

If used intentionally, it's a very damaging form of emotional abuse, and it's often done so surreptitiously that the target may not even be aware of it.

If you've ever heard phrases such as "I never said that", "you are imagining things", "you're too sensitive", "why are you making such a big deal out of this?" you've most likely been the target of gaslighting. It can happen in relationships, at work, and in society at large: Donald Trump's labeling of the media as "fake media" and creating his own form of reality is an example of gaslighting. Men finding excuses for their sexism is gaslighting: catcalling is a compliment, telling a woman to smile is harmless banter, calling homosexuals derogative terms is all in good fun, touching someone without consent is just being friendly, not taking no for an answer is being persistent (which is also a compliment, don't you know?), raping a woman who wore a short skirt or was drunk or went home with him meant she was asking for it.

If you're repeatedly being told by your parents that your fears are unreasonable, your frequent crying the behaviour of a drama queen and your need for extra reassurance attention-seeking, you believe them. And you believe that your needs are wrong and shameful and that you perceive the world and yourself not in the right way.

Being raised by a gaslighting caregiver has far-reaching repercussions: if your boss insists that they never said that even though you could have sworn they did, you believe them. After all, you have a history of getting things wrong, you must have gotten this one wrong as well.

If you confront a gaslighting partner about a lie you know they told and they turn it around and accuse you of making stuff up or that you're crazy, you are much more likely to believe them. Your parents said the same thing about you, surely they can't all be wrong?

Gaslighting is a horrible way of damaging a person's self-esteem and trust in themselves, and it's more common than you may think.

Talking about it with Tori is incredibly reassuring. I'm so relieved to hear that my emotions are valid and real, and even though learning that some people are purposely trying to mess with your head is sad, it's a great comfort to find out that I'm not the horrible person I was led to believe I am.

Another harmful lesson I learnt growing up was that I wasn't good enough the way I was. It taught me that I had to earn people's love and affection. I had to look a certain way, work hard, strive to always accomplish more, be nice and pleasant and uncomplicated. No messy display of emotions please! That shit was not meant for the public, you only did that far away from other eyes. My parents abhorred tears, PDA, and intimate confessions to other people. They were big fans of the stiff upper lip, being stoic, and keeping mushy feelings to oneself.

That's a very stressful way to live. What if you get sick, or lose your job, or gain thirty pounds? Does that mean you're worth less? Are people with disabilities automatically less worthy? What if you develop a round, comfortable belly? Or you have a mental breakdown, burnout, or quit your job because it's making you sick?

The answer to all these questions is obvious – of course you're not any less worthy – but in truth it's more complicated. Because all the conditioning starts when we are young, and a lot of it is happening on a subconscious level. If we are not aware of what we believe it's impossible to change. You can't change something you don't see.

You may know in theory that all human beings are inherently worthy, but if you grew up with conditional love, you believe you are different. Your experience has taught you that *you* have to work for love. It's a lonely and exhausting way to live, to be convinced that you have to work harder than anybody else to be deserving of love and respect.

Tori's lesson that beliefs are thoughts and that we can let go of them whenever we want is working for me this time. Once she unearths this conviction I wasn't even aware of, she tells me once more that I don't have to hang on to it if I don't want to. And wouldn't you know it, it works! I have no idea how, but once I *see* the subconscious bias I had against myself and compare it to what *I* believe about the worthiness of every single human being, I can release the old bias. It's amazing!

We use the same technique on something else that's been bothering me.

I tell Tori how I sometimes completely freak out when I come home, Richard isn't there and I don't know where he went. It's worth noting that we are not the kind of couple that's joined at the hip and does everything together. We don't know what the other is doing every second of the day because we trust each other, and we are independent people. I love that about our marriage.

But there are times when my common sense and reason have left the building. I'm transformed into a total wreck of frayed nerves and worst-case-scenarios, and I'm powerless to change that. When I'm in one of those episodes every little thing makes me go into a full-on panic. One of the biggest triggers is when he isn't home, and I can't get a hold of him. I'm convinced that something terrible has happened to him: he had a heart attack and lies somewhere on the ground, slowly dying; he got into a car accident; one of our horses or cows trampled him and he's bleeding out. Deep down I know that this is irrational and highly unlikely, but my entire being is panicking like it is real. My heart races, my breathing is shallow and ragged, I sweat and shake, and tears are blurring my eyes.

On more than one occasion I've called his buddies in a frenzy, asking if he's with them, trying unsuccessfully to keep the panic out of my voice. They are bewildered, because usually I come across as pretty chill (ha! If they only knew), and this behaviour is very unlike me.

Another time I mobilized our neighbours to help me search for him all over our ten-acre property because I was so sure that he was lying somewhere, gravely injured. In those moments I believe that I have a premonition, like when people tell you they just *knew* that their son was in danger, raced to his apartment and saved him from a suicide attempt.

If I'm having a premonition, don't look for him and he ends up dead, then his death is on me. It's a terrible ordeal to go through, and I'm always deeply ashamed afterwards.

After I've told Tori the sorry tale she says sympathetically: "You have killed your husband a thousand times. Don't you think that's enough?"

It sure is.

I know what's coming next, and I'm determined to give it my all. Come on Sedona Method, work your magic! Could I, would I, should I let it go? Yes, please! Right now if you don't mind.

It sort of works. I don't alert half the neighbourhood anymore when I can't find my husband. I tell myself that worrying doesn't help anything or anybody, least of all me. I do deep breathing exercises or take the dogs for a walk.

Have I transformed into a picture of serenity living in the now, being calm and collected? I wish.

Will I always worry about him dying before me? Yes I will. (A 25-year age difference will do that to a girl with anxiety.)

But I haven't had another one of those anxiety attacks, which is a huge win.

While Tori has helped me a lot, we have reached the end of our road together. I haven't had the courage to talk to her about my drinking, mostly because if she starts with the three questions again I'll scream. They don't work for everything, and I know they don't work for this (I tried).

The relationship between therapist and client is an intimate one. You have to trust your therapist implicitly, and even though I like her a lot, something isn't quite right. We are not as good a match as I hoped we would be.

It's like buying a dress that looks great, but that doesn't fit right. It's pinching under your armpits, and while you could ignore it because you look good in it, you know there is a better dress for you out there that won't pinch.

I thank her for everything she has done for me and tell her I can take it from here. I do feel a lot better equipped than I did before our time together.

Am I cured? Hell no. But I have a few more tools for my ongoing fight against my mental illness, and for that I'm grateful. I'm even hopeful that I've got it all figured out now! Well, that's a thought that I need to let go of, because as you will see, I couldn't be more wrong.

Another big whammy is patiently waiting for me, biding its time, getting ready to strike.

It will be here soon.

Puppies

Phew, all this stuff about depression and anxiety and COVID gets pretty depressing, doesn't it? I promised you some lighthearted stuff, and is there anything more lighthearted or life-affirming than puppies? No, there isn't. Enjoy the hell out of this chapter, because right after this we're moving on to the next catastrophe. Sorry guys, it wasn't my decision; that's how life has been the last few years. I should have named this book *A series of unfortunate events*, but that title was already taken.

Anyway, lean back and enjoy, because you are about to become part of one of the most joyful times of my life!

In September of 2020 we breed our big, beautiful Šarplaninac dog Teddy to our Great Pyrenees dog Pete. We happen to witness the act, and while I'm familiar with the humping part I didn't know that they stay stuck together for a while. Once he dismounts I expect him to happily trot off into the sunset, but he does not. Instead they stand next to each other, bums attached, smiling goofily with tongues lolling in postcoital bliss. I guess it's the doggy version of cuddling, and I'm here for it. They stay like this for fifteen minutes or so before separating and lying down for a well-deserved nap.

Unbeknownst to me, my go-big-or-go-home husband decides to breed our Blue Heeler Dixie at the same time. I don't notice that she's pregnant until she's halfway through her pregnancy when she's getting round, and her teats are starting to swell up. When I question the stupidity of his decision he says that "we're already getting one litter, a second one won't make a difference". Say what? Numbers don't matter? There's no difference between ten or twenty? Geez. But it's too late now, the train has left the station and all I can do is buckle up and wait for the puppy extravaganza.

Nine short weeks later Teddy gives birth to nine gorgeous, cinnamon-coloured puppies who look like little bear cubs. I marvel at the efficiency of canine procreation: 63 days and those puppies are fully cooked! Very impressive. Teddy's whelping box is in the barn, and I find all nine puppies already there one morning, but Dixie is giving birth in one of our bedrooms in a large crate. Four days after Teddy's pups are born we wake up and find Dixie moving around restlessly and sniffing between her hind legs frequently. It's time! At first we stick around, but we can tell that she wants to be left alone so we leave the room and quietly close the door.

"We're right outside if you need anything," I whisper, and I swear I can see her rolling her eyes, telling me in no uncertain terms that she got this.

Richard and I are pacing outside, straining our ears for any sound, but all is quiet. I didn't know what to expect, maybe some whining or panting? I press my ear against the door but there is no sound. When I can't stand the suspense for a moment longer I softly open the door and peek inside.

Dixie is lying in her crate, and she's not alone. "Rich, look!" I whisper-scream. "There are puppies!" He's right there behind me, with the same goofy smile on his face that I imagine I'm wearing. "Look at that," he smiles and takes a quick look at the three pups. "All healthy and looking good," he says, and then he gently shoos me out of the room. "I don't think she's done yet, give her some peace. She knows what she's doing."

He's right about that. By the end of the morning she has given birth to six perfect, black-and-white little puppies the size of guinea pigs, licked them dry and cleaned up the crate before we can give her a hand. It's incredible. The entire process is so clean, quick, and efficient, it's a miracle.

Now we have fifteen puppies, and I take back every unkind word I may have said to or about my husband in regard to having two litters at the same time. I'm in heaven! We have the six Blue Heeler/Border Collie puppies in the house and nine Šarplaninac/Great Pyrenees puppies in the barn, and I hang out with them whenever I can. Teddy and Dixie are both first-time mothers who excel at their new roles, and I can't get enough of watching them. I was expecting having to clean their boxes, but the mamas do it all: they lick their babies' tiny bottoms to encourage them to poop, and then they eat their poop, keeping everything meticulously clean. That's next level dedication!

The first two weeks the pups do nothing but nurse and sleep, and we have zero work with them. All we do is watch them grow, make sure the mamas eat enough to keep up with their offspring's ravenous appetite, and tell them several times a day what good moms they are. Just like with humans there are good and bad mothers in the animal world – not all mothers are automatically great. But our two are not only devoted mamas who look after their babies exceptionally well, they also don't mind my frequent visits.

By the end of week two the puppies have opened their eyes and ears and are starting to stand up. Things are about to get interesting!

We start feeding them by the end of week three when they're getting their first teeth to help the moms out. Teddy especially has her paws full feeding her nine hungry hippos and could use some help. We soak puppy food in warm water to make it nice and mushy, and once it's soft we present it to the puppies. They get it at once and start devouring it enthusiastically. We also move Dixie's babies out of the crate and into a swimming pool that we put up in our living room. Google has told us that this works, but the puppies must not have gotten the memo – the first one crawls over the edge and plops down on the other side of the pool within five minutes, soon followed by an adventurous brother. They're tottering around in front of the Christmas tree like the most adorable little drunks you've ever seen, and I'm so grateful for them that I tear up.

It's December of 2020, Christmas is cancelled due to all the COVID restrictions, the number of new cases is rising, but right now I don't care. Being with the dogs and puppies gives me a happiness and joy I haven't experienced all year.

Dogs have always saved me. No matter how dark the depression gets, how red-hot the rage of PMDD, how all-consuming the incessant worries of anxiety – my dogs will pull me out of it. There is no love like a dog's love. It's pure, truly unconditional, and contagious. Their joy of seeing you, of wanting to be with you every moment of every day, the exuberance with which they greet you even if you've only been gone ten minutes – it's the best feeling in the world.

Dogs are highly sensitive to their people's physical and mental health. When I'm going through a depressive episode, my corgi Lily won't leave my side, snuggling up close to me even though she isn't a snuggler. She senses that I'm vulnerable and looks out for me.

I have vivid, sometimes distressing dreams almost every night and moan and talk in my sleep. Dixie will wake me up when I get restless or distressed by crawling on top of me and licking my face. Feeling her warm, compact body on me grounds me like nothing else can. There's no room for nightmares with a dog right there; they chase all the bad thoughts away.

When I was younger I always wanted to have a girl posse. I dreamed of having a group of female BFFs, but it never quite penned out that way – mainly because I'm an introvert who prefers her own company to that of groups of people. But I didn't know anything about introverts and extroverts until I was in my thirties, so in my teens and twenties I was always conflicted about what I thought I wanted (being part of a large group) and what I truly craved. I'm telling you, awareness it's where it's at: you can't find true happiness until you know who you are and what makes you tick.

Once I figured out that I'm more of a one-on-one person I thought I'd have to bury my dreams of having a girl posse.

I couldn't have been more wrong. I've always had the most kickass entourage of badass bitches; I just didn't recognize it for a while. Lily, Dixie, and Teddy are my ride or die besties, and you can't ask for better company. They are always in an upbeat mood, there's never any drama, they are happy to see me every time, don't talk shit behind my back, and they know how to have a good time. They are the best friends a girl could wish for.

And now they have given me this amazing gift of fifteen exuberant little bundles of joy, and I didn't have to endure a single baby shower. (Baby showers and I don't get along.) Thanks ladies!

Everybody had warned me how much work puppies are, and at first I smugly thought that they were all wrong. They had either exaggerated wildly or didn't have mamas as efficient as ours. But around week four I have to admit that they weren't wrong after all. The pups are now fully mobile, they are eating like little machines, and what goes in has to come out. The amount of poop and pee these little creatures generate is astonishing. The nine big puppies are outside which helps a lot, but Dixie's six are in the living room.

We've replaced the swimming pool with an indoor playpen, and the sight that awaits me every morning is breathtaking. I mean that literally – I have to hold my breath as I get paper towels, a bucket with hot, soapy water, and a rag, open the playpen and let the little monsters out to clean up. There is poop *everywhere* inside the pen. It's a shitstorm of magnificent proportions – a shitstravaganza. While the pups are overjoyed to see me I'm scrubbing vigorously, mouth breathing only, peeling dried feces off the floor, and exchanging the soiled towels for clean ones, all the while fending off sharp little teeth that are digging painfully into my hands, arms, and legs. Yes, the teeth have come in, and they are weapons of skin destruction. I have scratch marks all over, neck and face included, because who can resist picking up a handful of puppies and letting them climb all over you? Not this girl. I can't get enough of them; teeth and excrements be damned. If dogs are good for one's soul, puppies have that effect about a thousandfold, which means this is one of the happiest times of my life. It's a lovefest, and I wish I could bottle up this feeling for a rainy day. Since that's not possible I take tons of videos and inhale their incomparable smell to ingrain it into my brain as deeply as possible. I never want to forget it.

We soon establish an assembly line of preparing puppy mush. We have to make several buckets daily to keep up with their ferocious appetites, especially for Teddy's big pups. They're now looking exactly like teddy bears come to life, and they are the cutest creatures you'll ever see. Every time we step outside they come running towards us in their adorably clumsy way, and soon you're surrounded by a sea of fur, all clamouring for scratches, snuggles, and food. Teddy has reached the stage where she doesn't want to nurse anymore, and who can blame her? I've felt those teeth, and you don't want them anywhere near a sensitive area like a nipple.

However, the pups don't give up easily, stalking her like crazed fans stalk their favourite celebrity, and she usually lets them nurse for a bit, standing there patiently with nine fluffballs lined up beneath her, little faces turned upwards, sucking greedily. That dog really has the patience of a saint.

Meanwhile, Dixie is going through the same inside the house. We let the puppies out of their playpen several times a day so they can play and roam around, and for me to clean it up. When we put them back inside Dixie usually goes in with them for a bit to nurse and settle them down before we let her out. If we're not quick enough she simply climbs over the playpen for a much-deserved nap away from her babies.

I couldn't have dreamed of a better way to end the most bizarre year of our lives. After ten months of fear, uncertainty, drastic changes to everyday life and an overuse of the word "unprecedented" these fifteen puppies have refilled my happiness reserves. They are overflowing, and I'm positively brimming with anticipation for the new year. The vaccine is here, ready to come out any day now, and carries with it the promise of life returning to some semblance of normalcy. Work will become easier, people will stop dying, and we may even be able to see each other again!

New life brings new hope, and my hope is multiplied by fifteen. As I'm holding armfuls of puppies with a permanent smile on my face I'm certain that the worst year in living history is behind us.

Little do I know that it's about to get much worse.

Great Expectations

The new year dawns with a huge amount of expectation on everybody's part. We collectively hope that 2021 means the end of the pandemic and the return of all the big and little things we used to take for granted but have come to recognize for what they are: precious gifts. People dream of being able to go to concerts, sports events, vacations, the gym, or simply down the wrong way in the grocery store without being yelled at. Remember a time before all the arrows and Plexiglas and six-feet distance stickers on the floors everywhere? Ahh, the beauty of simpler times. We didn't appreciate how good we had it.

Hospital workers everywhere dream of a lightening of the crushing burden of too many sick and dying patients, of not having to change in and out of PPE dozens of times a day, and of giving our cracked and bleeding hands a break from constantly using hand sanitizer. We don't even dare hope that there might come a time where we can see each other's, or patients' faces again – we're resigned to the fact that we will have to wear masks at our workplace forever. But it would be nice to not have the crushing fear that seeing someone's exposed face might kill you and getting vaccinated is the key to that. My friend and I get the call that we can get our first dose in Lytton on January 25, and we jump at the chance. It's a joyful and emotional day and surely the beginning of the end, right?

But instead of getting easier, work is getting more heartbreaking. One of the terrible consequences of COVID is the neglect of all other diseases. Surgeries are still being cancelled, sick patients sent home to make room for sicker COVID patients, and most people can't see their doctors in person and are too afraid to come to the hospital out of fear of getting infected. As a result some people are getting diagnosed late – sometimes too late.

I come face to face with one such case.

On a Saturday morning I'm getting called in to the hospital to do a chest x-ray on a patient who is short of breath. She's a cheerful elderly woman who apologizes as soon as she lays eyes on me.

"I'm so sorry you have to come in, I'm sure it's nothing!" she says to me.

"Nonsense, that's what I'm here for," I assure her, adding with a wink, "I'm not doing it for free, you just made me money!"

She laughs, and we chat about the British royal family because she shares her first name with one of their prominent members. We continue our pleasant conversation as I process the first image, but what I see makes my heart plummet.

There's something big in her chest that doesn't belong there. I stare at it for a moment, dumbfounded, before continuing my small talk, now with a forced smile instead of a genuine one. I can't let on that anything is wrong because we are not allowed to make any comment whatsoever on what we see. If the patient asks we have to tell them to wait for the doctor to talk to them. Luckily she doesn't ask me, and as soon as I'm finished with her exam I return her to the emergency department.

I go straight to the nurse's station where the doctor is sitting on his computer. "Can you take a look at her chest x-ray right away?" I ask him. "There is something on it." He obliges, and I stand over him as he pulls up the images on the screen. As soon as he sees them, our eyes meet in mutual horrified understanding.

On my way out of the hospital I catch a glimpse of the doctor, the patient and her husband in the private consultation room that's reserved for breaking bad news.

Usually I wouldn't have any idea what's going on with a patient. We don't get to know the diagnosis, let alone the treatment plan or anything else. Our job is mainly that of a photographer – we take pictures of bones and that's that.

But over the next few weeks I x-ray her every weekend I am working. She keeps coming to the emergency department because her condition is rapidly deteriorating. Every time I see her she is as positive and kind as the first time I met her, but her body is wasting away. She grows weaker with each passing week. Bound by the invisible rules of our positions, we never mention what's going on, but we both know.

She dies three months after I took that initial x-ray, and I cry when I find out. I don't often get that close to patients, and it's hitting me hard. When I see her husband shortly after her death, I'm unable to say more than "I'm so sorry" – the most inadequate words in the English language when you try to express your condolences. Why don't we learn what to say in these situations? Death is the one common denominator that unites us all, yet we are not taught how to deal with it in our society.

Sadly, this is not the only case. My colleagues and I see more advanced cancers than ever before, often due to the fact that the patients couldn't see their doctor or didn't seek help early enough out of fear of getting COVID.

One day I x-ray a patient's ankle. He has told his doctor over the phone that it is "red and painful", so the doctor ordered an x-ray. As soon as the patient takes off his sock I know that something is very wrong. That ankle looks *angry*. It's bright red and radiates so much heat, you can practically see it coming off the leg in waves. The redness is wide-spread – how wide I don't know, because it disappears under his pant leg. I take the pictures, and when I'm done I tell him that he should go to the emergency department to see a doctor.

"Ahh, do I have to? I'd rather go home and wait for my doc to call me. He said he'd do it tomorrow," the patient says.

I throw caution to the wind. I'm not supposed to do what I'm about to, but he leaves me no choice. It's after hours, the doctor isn't in his office anymore for me to consult with, and I have a strong hunch that this is serious. "You have a bad infection, you *have* to get it looked at today," I urge him. When he still hesitates I add: "Tomorrow could be too late." I have no idea if that's true, but it does the trick; he agrees and wanders off to the ER.

Weeks later one of my co-workers tells me that the patient collapsed in the waiting room – he was in the beginning stages of sepsis. Sepsis, the body's extreme response to an infection, triggers a chain reaction in the body that will shut down the organs and lead to death if not treated promptly. The patient was treated in time, but who knows what could have happened if he had waited another day?

The heaviness of bearing witness to the worst news weighs me down. I seem to have lost the balance between being compassionate and detached, which is vital for healthcare workers to stay healthy. Instead I feel every bad news deeply, often having to fight back tears, hating the helplessness and the heavy emotions. Why can't I just shake it off like Taylor Swift tells us to? Why does it feel like it's happening to me? Am I that self-obsessed that I make their tragedy about myself? What is wrong with me?

In April, we are put on evacuation alert due to a nearby wildfire. A wildfire in April? This is highly unusual. It is suspected to be human-caused, and thanks to a combination of wind, drier than normal undergrowth and unseasonably warm weather there is a chance that it may come dangerously close to our house. I don't even know what "evacuation alert" means, but the Internet tells me that we have to be ready to leave our home on short notice. They recommend having an overnight bag ready with essential medication, a change of clothing, and copies of all our important documents. It seems like an overreaction since everything looks calm, aside from a tiny bit of smoke on the horizon that appears to be reassuringly far away. I drive past the wildfire area every day on my way to work, and you can barely see it from the road.

When I show up at work the day of the evacuation alert everybody expresses their astonishment that I'm there and not at home, packing. *Should* I be at home, packing? What's the right thing to do? This is yet another unprecedented time, and frankly, I'm sick of them. How about a nice long stretch of precedented times, please?

I stay at work, because Richard is home and will call me as soon as something changes. I also download an app that will alert you when there are emergency situations in your area, such as wildfires, floods, tornadoes, or other catastrophes.

I get my first notification from it a few days later when the evacuation alert is rescinded, and I sincerely hope that this will be the last time I hear its high-pitched sound.

It won't be.

In May, my friend Christina and I get our second COVID vaccine. We go once again to Lytton where the clinic is being held at the community hall. A bunch of hot young men – our guess is firefighters – are there to hand out snacks, bottles of water and juice boxes, and to lend a helping hand should anyone feel faint or get an adverse reaction after the shot. Hm, do I suddenly feel in need of some assistance? I rein in my spontaneous cougar impulse and accept a juice box instead. I haven't had one of those since I was in Elementary school, and I enjoy the three-and-a-half sips of sugary goodness (those juice boxes are *tiny*).

Afterwards we celebrate our fully vaccinated status by getting Chinese takeout. We eat our food next to a marker that proclaims Lytton as "the hottest spot in Canada".

We have no idea how terribly true this marker will turn out to be.

A couple of weeks later, over 200 unmarked graves are found with the help of ground-penetrating radar near the former Kamloops Indian Residential School. The remains are from children, some as young as three years old, and the shocking discovery makes news around the world.

Residential schools are a terrible part of Canada's history. Canada's first prime minister, John A. Macdonald, said the following in an 1883 speech to the House of Commons:

"When the school is on the reserve, the child lives with its parents, who are savages; he is surrounded by savages, and though he may learn to read and write his habits, and training and mode of thought are Indian. He is simply a savage who can read and write. It has been strongly pressed on myself, as the head of the Department, that Indian children should be withdrawn as much as possible from the parental influence, and the only way to do that would be to put them in central training industrial schools where they will acquire the habits and modes

of thought of white men."[8]

That's the reason for the residential schools. The Canadian government established a system of boarding schools whose primary goal was to "kill the Indian in the child", and whose terrifying reign lasted until 1996. For over one hundred years, more than 150,000 First Nations, Métis and Inuit children were placed in residential schools, often against the parents' will. Their hair was cut off, they were forbidden from speaking their language or practicing their cultural traditions, and they were given new names or even worse, just a number. Siblings were not allowed to speak to each other, and all noncompliance with the rules was severely punished. The underfunded schools, run by various churches, were in terrible condition: the buildings were drafty, the windows locked, and there were no fire escapes. The mortality rate was far above average compared to other schools, with many children dying of infectious diseases such as tuberculosis, smallpox, measles, or influenza; in fires; from poor nutrition caused by spoiled and insufficient food; suicide; or abuse. Some children were buried in unmarked graves such as the ones found in Kamloops; others were reported missing.

Sexual, emotional, and physical abuse was widespread, and the children had nobody they could confide in. They knew implicitly that they were not to tell anyone about what was going on at school, or about the deaths they witnessed.

Despite the approximately 80,000 residential school survivors who are still alive today, this piece of Canadian history is not well known, at least not in detail. While most people are vaguely aware of the existence of residential schools, they don't want to know what exactly happened there.

The non-Indigenous community would prefer to simply forget about it, to act like it happened a long time ago (it didn't; the last school closed in 1996) and that it wasn't that bad (it was worse).

But the discovery of dead children is impossible to ignore, especially when you live and work in communities where many people went through the

---

[8] Historica Canada, Residential Schools in Canada, http://education.historicacanada.ca/files/1 03/ResidentialSchools_Printable_Pages.pdf

experience themselves. It opens up old wounds, and the collective grief is palpable.

At the time of this writing, the exact number of unmarked graves is unknown. More and more unmarked graves are being found; the number is in the thousands. To make it even worse, there is evidence that some children's bodies were disposed of in lakes, rivers, and incinerators. Those bodies will never be found, and we will never know the true extent of the atrocities that were committed.

The reminder of how truly horrendous humans can treat their fellow human beings is unwelcome and heartbreaking. In the face of so much suffering, is it any wonder that we get depressed and hopeless?

In June we're getting an intense heat wave. At first I'm overjoyed. I love summer, and this dry heat is incredible! I head to the nearby river with the dogs every afternoon for a dip, reveling in the fact that the river is warm enough in June to sit in. There's a spot with a counter current that reminds me of the wild water channel at the public pool my sister and I went to as kids. We loved it when they turned on the jets and turned the lazy river into a foaming, exhilarating wild water adventure. This natural counter current gives me the same thrill and makes me miss my sister.

One day on my way home from work the thermometer in my car shows 48 degree Celsius, which is a temperature I have never experienced in my life. I pull over, turn off the car with its delicious air conditioning, and open the car door. The heat hits me like I've walked against a wall. It feels solid, like something I should be able to touch. I get out and slowly walk around, feeling as if I'm walking in a fire. There's no humidity so it's not soupy, but it feels unnatural. Wrong somehow, like it shouldn't exist. 48 degrees is not normal, at least not here, and certainly not in June. It gives me an uneasy feeling.

On Tuesday, June 29, Lytton records the hottest temperature in Canadian history: 49.6 degrees Celsius, 121.3 degrees Fahrenheit. It's hotter than Las Vegas has ever been, hotter than *anywhere* in Europe or South America. Let that sink in for a moment: Lytton, which is covered in snow several months every year, is hotter than Greece, Rio de Janeiro, or the Amazon jungle. It breaks its own temperature record three days in a row, just a few months after I was standing in a blizzard in its picturesque snow-covered streets.

And then June 30 dawns. The residents of Lytton prepare for another punishingly hot day. Most stay indoors close to the AC, chugging water and hoping for the heatwave to break. Many also keep an eye on the sky because a wildfire has been burning north of the town for several days, and they're keeping track of the smoke, worried it may move closer.

But that's not where the danger lies. Unbeknownst to them, a second fire has started to the south by the rail trestle, and in the afternoon, during the hottest and most stupefying time of day, hell descends upon Lytton. Seemingly out of nowhere, black, billowing smoke followed by a wall of fire tears through town, blown in by strong winds of up to 70km/h. It happens so fast that most residents don't have time to grab anything but their keys – they run for their lives with their clothes on their backs. Within fifteen minutes, the entire town burns; after thirty, 90% of Lytton is destroyed.

The residents have scattered, seeking refuge with friends and family or in the hastily thrown together emergency centers in the surrounding communities. The next day is Canada Day, a national holiday. It's usually a favourite of Canadians that's being celebrated with barbecues, parades, concerts, and fireworks. But this year, some celebrations have been cancelled after the recent gruesome discovery of the unmarked graves, and now an entire town has burnt to the ground in a matter of minutes.

Canada Day is cancelled for many of us.

All day Christina and I text each other photos, memories, and expressions of our disbelief and sorrow.

The hospital we both worked at – gone.

The community hall where we got our second vaccine – gone.

The Chinese restaurant we both loved so much – gone.

The stone marker that proclaims Lytton to be "the hottest spot in Canada" must still be there, buried in soot and ash, a charred reminder of the hideous "honour" of being one of the hottest places on earth.

We had such great expectations for 2021, but they have gone up in flames. As it turns out, they are not the only ones – our beautiful province of British Columbia follows suit.

BC is on fire.

Surrounded by Fire

The fire that burnt Lytton to the ground – soon known as the Lytton Creek Fire – hasn't burnt itself out. On the contrary, the little town was just the appetizer, and it is ravenous for more. It grows at a rapid rate, the bone-dry woods nothing but kindling to feed its insatiable hunger, and worst of all, it is soon joined by other fires that spring up all over the province like mushrooms. Not even three weeks after one state of emergency has been lifted for BC (the one for COVID-19), another one is being declared on July 20 for the threat hundreds of wildfires pose to the people and properties of the Interior. Thousands of people are evacuated already, and tens of thousands are on evacuation alert. Fire fighters arrive from other provinces and Mexico to help the severely overworked local fire departments.

Our beautiful blue sky is being obscured by thick smoke, casting everything into a sepia light that gives it a fitting apocalyptic atmosphere. The sun hangs blood-red in the sky, emitting its deadly heat day in and day out, turning the grass, shrubs and trees into explosive tinderboxes that need nothing more than a hot glance to burst into flames. The air quality is so poor that children, the elderly, and anybody with breathing problems are advised to stay indoors with the windows closed. We are getting an influx of patients with respiratory problems in the hospitals, caused by the permanent smoke inhalation. Oh, and did I mention COVID? It's still alive and kicking, filling up our ICU beds and emergency rooms and depleting our already low energy and staffing reserves. We are losing people daily to evacuations, getting sick and getting burnt out, which leads to even more severe staffing shortages. It makes each of us question for how much longer we will be able to hang on before we are too exhausted to continue.

One of the nurses I work with has an experience so frightening, I can't believe she's still standing upright, let alone continuing to work.

Her home is built at the edge of a forest. For days she and her family watch with growing concern as the plume of smoke keeps moving closer. They cut down trees and dig trenches around the perimeter of their house to create a line the fire hopefully won't be able to cross. They also prepare for the worst and buy a generator, pump, and fire hoses, set everything up and fervently pray that they won't need to use any of it.

No such luck. The fire fighters that have been working nearby, fighting to hold the fire back knock on their door one day and inform them that they have to evacuate.

"You're staying though, right?" the husband asks.

"No sir, it's too dangerous. If the fire comes any closer it will cut off the only route of egress. We are leaving and so should you." Husband and wife look at each other. If they leave now their house will burn down. They will lose everything they have built together, everything they have worked so hard to create. It will be gone in minutes.

They thought they had prepared for this moment, but they realize in an instant that you can never truly prepare for anything like this. Now that it's upon them, the decision they have to make is paralyzing them.

However, there's no time to be paralyzed. They can see the fire coming down the hill, moving towards them fast. The fire trucks are leaving in a cloud of dust, the warnings of the fire chief still ringing in their ears.

"Take the kids and go," the husband tells his wife. He's made his decision.

She gives him a quick, hard hug. "Stay safe and don't do anything stupid," she whispers into his ear, and then she quickly turns away so he can't see the tears in her eyes.

The husband and his friends save their home. Incredibly, while this is going on, the wife still continues to show up for her 12-hour shifts, caring for others while going through an unbelievably stressful time herself. She does it because she knows that if she doesn't come to work, there will be nobody else to take her place. She does it for her co-workers and her community. She does it because she is a deeply compassionate and caring woman.

But she shouldn't have to be in this situation. She should be at home with her kids and her husband, recovering after one of the scariest and most traumatizing experiences of her life.

She is putting her own health at risk in the service of others. How much are we expected to sacrifice for our jobs?

In August it's my husband's and my turn.

It's the weekend and I'm on call, staying at the staff house 100 kilometers away from home. The drive to and from work has been treacherous over the last six weeks, with highways frequently being closed on short notice due to wildfires burning right alongside them. There are only two direct routes I can take plus one that's a two-hour detour, and each one of these roads has been closed in turn. My biggest fear is that they will all be closed at the same time, leaving me stranded and cut off from home. It hasn't happened yet, but the fires are burning ever closer, having now reached a total number of 1,600 fires across the province.

On Sunday morning at 11:39 I get the phone call from Richard I've been expecting and dreading since June 30. "The smoke is getting really bad here and it's extremely windy. You better come home."

I still have 20 hours left of being on call. But when I talk to the hospital staff and tell them that it looks like we are about to be evacuated, all they say is "we understand. Go home and save your animals".

I tear through the staff house, packing my stuff, with tears running down my cheeks and panic threatening to overwhelm me. "Calm down, it's gonna be okay," I chant under my breath, forcing myself to take deep, yogic breaths. The breaths help, the chant doesn't. What if I don't make it home in time? What if the fire actually reaches us? What is gonna happen to our animals? We have horses, sheep, cows, dogs, cats, and birds – it would take at least a full day to evacuate them all. And where to? The fire has surrounded us, nobody knows where safety is.

The two direct routes are both closed so I have to take the long one home. I have horror visions that it might get closed as well, and my panic makes me clumsy and slow. Richard calls again and reminds me to drive carefully and to take my time. "Don't rush, keep at the speed limit!" he says with concern in his voice. I promise that I will and white-knuckle it home.

It's just after 2pm when I arrive, the sky an orange-brown and the sun a hazy red disc that's barely visible. The wind is whipping my hair crazily around my head and there's smoke everywhere. The wind is blowing the Lytton Creek Fire that has now destroyed over 50,000 hectares directly towards us.

I jump out of the car with my arms full and race into the house. Where to start? For a long moment I stand immobile, unable to decide what to do first. I drop everything on the floor, sink to my knees and burst into tears again. The dogs snuggle close, licking my face, and for a few minutes I stay there, crying and stroking their soft coats. "Okay team," I eventually say out loud. "First things first: laundry."

Doing laundry might seem irrational at this moment (why wash clothes that might burn up in a few hours?), but you do strange things when you're scared out of your mind. I've always found doing laundry relaxing, and it calms me down enough to make a plan.

Once the washing machine is running, I get my suitcase out of the basement and start filling it with our important papers, passports, laptop, medication, my camera, and other bits and pieces I want to keep.

I pack a second suitcase with toiletries, clothes, dog and cat food.

Richard is outside doing chores, making his own list. We move a trailer load of hay and Richard's tractor to a friend's place. I save files from my desktop computer to an external drive. The road leading out of our subdivision is packed with neighbours hauling out boats, trailers, dirt bikes, quads, and whatever else they want to save. Where are they hauling it to? I have no idea. All major highways leading out of the danger zone are closed; there is only one route left. If that one gets shut down, we will be cut off from the rest of the world.

Nobody knows where the illusive safe spot is, but the panic is contagious, so everybody is moving stuff *somewhere*.

And then the car is packed, and we wait. It's still windy and smoky, and the sky is getting dark, almost black. It looks like a storm is coming, and the atmosphere is loaded with an almost tangible threat. We keep looking at the horizon, checking for flames, texting friends to find out if they have heard anything. "Do you know where the fire is? How far away? Is it coming? Will we have to leave?"

Eventually darkness falls, and there it is: the tell-tale red glow. I get a text from a friend living not far from us: "The order just came in: we are getting evacuated."

Shortly after I get the official update on my phone, and soon after that the police cars are making their way up the hill, knocking on peoples' doors to tell them to get out.

"What are we gonna do?" I whisper.

"Let's wait and see," Richard replies.

We watch the procession of trucks and trailers snake slowly down the hill, followed by the police cars with their red and blue flashing lights.

And then it's just us. We silently watch the red glow veering off to the side and bypassing us, heading directly towards town. Merritt is being put on evacuation alert within the hour, with the burning hills surrounding it painting the black night red.

At around midnight I fall asleep, emotionally drained, but Richard stays up to keep watch until dawn.

The next morning dawns bright and with a clear sky. We can see the blue of the sky for the first time in a week! Everything is calm, the air is fresh and clean.

There's no sign of fire or smoke, and the best part: it's cool and around midday it's starting to rain. Hallelujah!

Over the next few hours we connect with friends and neighbours, learning where everybody ended up. Most ranchers and people with livestock have stayed behind to look after their animals. Others have spray-painted their names and telephone numbers onto their horses' sides or written them with Sharpie on their hooves and let them go, hoping they will find a safe spot and water on their own.

The rodeo grounds in Merritt have been transformed into an impromptu animal shelter, with many people sleeping in their RVs and campers to stay close to and care for their animals.

What will happen if Merritt is also being evacuated? Nobody knows. Every last hotel, motel, and B&B is filled to capacity with refugees from other communities. Some people had to move from one emergency centre to the next as each is forced to move out of the way of the insatiable fire.

The main highway leading to Chilliwack, the city designated as next emergency centre, is closed due to – you guessed it – yet another fire. There is only one last road left to get there, a detour that's choked with traffic causing huge delays.

There are 24/7-roadblocks preventing people to return home unless they have a special permit, which also means that we can't leave. That puts us into an oddly tranquil bubble for the five days the evacuation lasts. We can't go anywhere or do anything, so I get to sit down and exhale. The weather continues to cooperate by being cool and rainy, the air remains clear and the sky a greyish blue, providing us with a sense of safety and peace like nothing else has during this terrible summer.

We receive countless phone calls from concerned friends with offers of help and shelter, and they mean the world to us. The solidarity we collectively experienced a year and a half ago at the beginning of the pandemic is making a short comeback, and it's incredibly reassuring to see. Faith in humanity: restored (if only briefly, but we'll get to that shortly).

After five days, the evacuation is suddenly over. Without any warning we get the all-clear, and shortly after, our neighbours return in a procession of cars, trailers, and RVs. Two days later, I return to work. Nothing happened to us, we are the lucky ones, why wouldn't I?

One of my regular routes to work is open again, and I drive through a changed landscape. The formerly green trees are reduced to black, charred sticks. I pass by burnt down barns and ranches who lost cattle in the fires. I try not to imagine their blackened bodies and fail. Some trees are still smoking slightly, making me feel nervous. Is it going to start again? The whole scene reminds me powerfully of the part in *The Hunger* Games where Katniss returns to the destroyed District 12. Just like in the movie it looks like a war happened here, and in a way it did. I'm not sure who won.

My heart is heavy as I drive past the destruction, but then it lifts and I laugh out loud: the herd of wild sheep is standing on the road as if nothing happened, as unimpressed as always by my approaching car. I roll down my window and greet them enthusiastically. "Hi guys, you made it! You clever creatures. The fire couldn't get you down, could it? You have no idea how happy I am to see you!"

They ignore me and take their sweet time to slowly move out of the way. I could kiss them.

Nature has a way of teaching us resilience like nothing else can. Just a few weeks after the devastation of the fire, the blackness of the scorched ground is covered in fresh green grass. New life is rising from the ashes, demonstrating that life goes on. What has been destroyed can be rebuilt, new trees will replace the old ones, and the animals return from where they have been hiding to resume life like before.

The only thing that can't be replaced is lost lives. As summer turns into fall, the fourth COVID wave wreaks havoc in the hospitals. The Delta variant, more contagious than the previous variants, leads to severe illness in unvaccinated people and has filled up our hospital beds once again. After a year and a half of living and working in the pandemic, after just having survived a harrowing summer of more uncertainty and fear, hospital workers are at a breaking point.

And what we wake up to on September 1, 2021, manages to finally break some of us.

Protests

As soon as I walk into the hospital on September 1 I know something's up. There's a weird vibe, and I beeline to one of my favourite nurses, Nina, to find out what's going on.

"There's a walkout planned today for one o'clock," she tells me worriedly.

"What do you mean, a walkout?" I have no idea what she's talking about.

She pulls up something on her phone and holds it out to me. It's a flyer that announces a "World Wide Walkout" in large letters, and in smaller print underneath "Health Freedom: Stand up for freedom now or lose everything". The flyer continues: "Vaxxed or unvaxxed, masked or unmasked, all are welcome. It's time!! Stand together, reject the tyranny of mandatory vaccines." Next to it there's a list of locations in all ten provinces where the walkouts will take place, and when I read it I look up in disbelief.

"It's happening in front of hospitals? Why?"

Nina shakes her head in disgust. "It's organized by a group that calls itself *Canadian Frontline Nurses*. They're protesting against the mandatory vaccine for healthcare workers and the vaccine passport, and they want us to leave our jobs today at 1pm. Can you imagine? What nurse would leave her patients to protest against something that saves lives? They are nuts."

I stare at her, speechless. I feel like I've been hit in the stomach. At last I find my voice again. "Do you think they will protest here?"

She shrugs her shoulders. "I have no idea. Nobody from this hospital will "walk out", but I know a few people in town who are against the vaccine. They might just be insensitive enough to show up and give us a hard time. I hope not, but it's possible. Don't go outside at 1, just in case."

I walk back to my department, feeling a crushing mix of disgust, apprehension, worry, and sadness. It's just after 8 am, five hours before the protests are scheduled to happen, and all we can do is wait and hope that no-one will show up. In the meantime I google the so-called *Canadian Frontline Nurses*.

The group was founded by two nurses from Ontario who first were members of the *Global Frontline Nurses*(GFN). GFN is a conspiracy group spouting false theories about COVID "fraud" and claiming hospitals are lying about the pandemic.

Both nurses have participated in rallies against lockdowns and wearing masks and flew to Washington, D.C. on January 6, 2021, to speak at an anti-lockdown rally on the steps of Capitol Hill hours before thousands of Trump supporters stormed the Capitol to stop the certification of the presidential election results.

They have since been fired from their jobs, which speaks volumes. The majority of healthcare workers who have worked with COVID patients is pro-vaccine. It's a protection we have been desperate for in 2020, when all that stood between us and a deadly virus was a flimsy piece of fabric. We've seen firsthand the positive difference the vaccine makes not only in the severity of the disease (vaccinated people rarely die of COVID), but also in the treatment of patients with other diseases. The more people are vaccinated, the less patients need to be hospitalized for COVID, which finally makes desperately needed room for other patients who have been neglected for the past year and a half.

It's inappropriate and highly misleading for that group of conspiracy freaks to call themselves nurses, because they do not represent the values of nursing nor the majority of healthcare workers. To make matters worse, that title gives a wrong impression to the public, making it sound like we don't believe in the science of vaccines which leads to uncertainty and spreads fear and confusion.

I close the website about the *Canadian Frontline Nurses* with disgust and hope that nothing will happen at one o'clock.

That hope proves to be futile.

Later that day I watch in horror as thousands of protesters gather in front of many major hospitals in Canada with signs comparing the **choice** of not getting vaccinated with the persecution and murder of Jews during the Holocaust. I see a white woman holding a sign stating that "segregation and medical coercion are a violation of basic human rights" – a statement that's 100% correct but used so brutally out of context that it's shockingly insensitive. How can you compare racial segregation with some minor inconveniences for a limited time for a **choice** *you* made out of your own free will?

What's so horrible about these protests is not the fact that people are against the vaccine passport or vaccines in general. I know that there is always more than one way of looking at something. As long as there are people there will be differing opinions, and that's how it should be. Every topic has supporters and opponents.

What upsets me and my co-workers so much is the fact that they have chosen *hospitals* as their venue for protesting. Not city hall where the decisions are made, or a big open space where they are not blocking traffic or upsetting patients and frontline workers. They have chosen the place where the war is being fought, largely unseen by the public since the dying literally happens in isolation.

They are attacking the people who are risking their lives to help their communities, some of whom have spent months away from their children, parents, and grandparents to not expose them to the virus.

They are figuratively (and in some instances, literally) spitting in our faces, calling us gullible *sheeples* who have been brainwashed by the government, while we look on from windows where patients behind us are dying horrendous deaths all alone. Elderly patients with dementia get agitated by the loud honking outside. Family members of patients who are ill or dying are brought to tears as they have to pass through the noisy protesters, most of whom don't wear masks.

The biggest problem about COVID is that most of the public has only seen easy cases. The neighbour who got it but "didn't feel worse than having a cold", the asymptomatic friend who "felt totally fine, dude", the random Facebook person who claims they "had it really bad" but recovered just fine.

They have no idea what happens behind the closed doors of the ICU. Here's what it looks like:

A 39-year-old formerly healthy patient who had to be put into a medically induced coma in order to survive.

Patients who have such intense pain with every breath they take, they describe it "like a thousand bees are stinging the insides of my chest".[9]

Patients who are begging their nurses to put them out of their misery, because they have the worst headache of their lives, they're more isolated than they've ever been due to isolation restrictions, and they have given up hope of ever recovering.

Patients who feel like they're being smothered.

Patients who have a fever so high, they feel like they're on fire.

Patients who have delirium, which makes them severely disoriented, confused, and panicky.

Patients who feel like they're running a marathon while breathing through the smallest straw imaginable. They cannot catch their breath, so they panic, which makes them hyperventilate, which makes them even less capable of catching their breath – until they feel like they're drowning. But they're not quite drowning, because as awful as drowning is, at least it's fast.

COVID isn't. You might be drowning for days, until you either die, or you get intubated. Intubation is the process where a tube is inserted through the mouth into the airway. The tube is connected to a machine that pumps air into the lungs. As you can imagine, this procedure is so invasive and uncomfortable that the patient needs to be heavily sedated. The lucky ones who survive often say afterwards that they don't remember the ordeal, which is probably for the best. While procedures like intubation save lives, they can also be traumatizing to patients. If you get to pick between wearing a mask or having to go through an invasive, violent procedure, I know which one I'd choose.

We understand that everybody is tired of the pandemic and the restrictions.

---

[9] Vox, What it's like to die from Covid-19, https://www.vox.com/2021/2/20/22280817/covid-19-deaths-us-nursing-home-icu-ventilator

We healthcare workers are collectively more tired than we've ever been in our lives. But what feels like a giant slap in the face is being mocked and assaulted for doing our jobs. We know that we will see some of the people who have attended today's protests, unmasked and unvaccinated, in our hospitals soon. And we will do what we've signed up to do: we will take care of them. We will hold their hand, hold their puke-bucket, listen to their fears and regrets.

We will do everything in our power to help.

Except that some of us won't be there anymore. Some of us will have left by then, unable to take the stress and abuse any longer. When we chose our careers we were prepared for long hours, working nights and weekends and holidays, for seeing pain and hardship. What we weren't prepared for is being labelled "enforcers of slavery" or being accused of "conducting human experimentation". We weren't prepared to be kicked in the groin for caring.

It feels as if we have fallen down Alice's rabbit hole and everything is turned upside down. What is right and good has suddenly been twisted into the opposite, and what's saving lives – vaccines – has been turned into a weapon. The protesters use the weapon against us healthcare workers, but also unknowingly against themselves and their fellow men: they will kill people who are unsure and easily swayed by making them believe that what they have to fear is the very thing that could save their lives. The beds in the ICUs are filled with patients who are dying of COVID, and they are almost exclusively unvaccinated.

We are witnesses who see it, breathe it, work with it and are around it every day.

But now we are being called liars, and by the time these protesters see the truth – when they or someone they love gets deadly ill – it will be too late. Most of us will still be there to do our best to help them and ease their suffering – but not all of us. It will have broken some of us.

While September 1 was a dark day, September 2 is much brighter. As we suspected, the protesters from the day before represent a loud but small minority. Most people stand behind healthcare workers, and they're showing their support by dropping off cards or gifts and offering words of love and appreciation. It's a gesture that's spirit-saving and incredibly important to everyone's morale. It keeps us going when we want to give up and reminds us that our patients still need us.

I'm a mess though. I haven't slept properly in two months, I'm losing hair due to stress, and I have a potbelly that's either from too much wine or perimenopause, and I don't know which option is worse. All I know is that I need help, and the only help I can think of is therapy. Even though I didn't exactly love it last time it was illuminating and helpful. Besides, I'm desperate, and I have no idea what else to do.

It's time to face my demons again.

Therapy II

"What causes depression?"

It's my second session with my new therapist. Lola is young, cheerful, exuberant, and full of energy. She's also quite different to Tori. During our first session I gave her an expert rundown of my mental illness, feeling smug about being an old hand at this therapy thing. I was ready to launch into my childhood and how everything can be blamed on it, but to my surprise her focus is not on the past; it's on the present.

She gently guides me towards mindfulness, which she defines as paying attention to and focusing on the present moment, not the past or future. She also talks about the attitude that will benefit us best, one where we are compassionate observers instead of being judgmental and becoming too emotional.

I'm digging all this. When I tell her that my guiding word for the year is mindfulness, she claps her hands with excitement and beams. "I love our alignment!" she tells me, and so do I. Our connection is instantaneous and effortless, and talking to her feels like talking to a friend.

She teaches me about self-compassion, something many women lack, and about human giver syndrome, something women have way too much of. Human giver syndrome is a term that was coined by sisters Emily and Amelia Nagoski in their book *Burnout*, and it describes the unspoken expectation of women to give everything to others. From the moment we are born we are given the role to care and nurture without complaint, and to put ourselves last. Little girls are much more often given the responsibility to look after younger siblings than little boys, because it's assumed that we are all born with the need to mother others.

Self-care is considered selfish and heartless. Human giver syndrome is the foundation of the belief that women should do childcare and housework on top of having jobs – it's "in their genes" to do these things and is seen as part of their female identity and responsibility.

But I digress, which incidentally will happen often during our sessions. Lola is a feminist and passionate about helping women take better care of themselves, and she awakens something in me that I didn't realize was there. It's a seed that has been dormant my entire life, patiently waiting for sun and water, and she is giving me that sun and water. The seed is waking up and starting to sprout.

Now I'm eagerly waiting for an answer to my question about what causes depression. I've been wondering about that for a while. My sweet family doctor had told me all those years ago that it was simply a chemical imbalance in my brain, and that answer was exactly what I wanted to hear at the time: he converted my mental problem into a physical one that I could take a pill for. Perfect! But I have since learnt that it's not that straightforward, and my own experience has proven that. If it was, taking my antidepressants would have cured my mental illness, and it clearly hasn't.

So what is it then?

Lola considers the question for a moment before answering. "It's a combination of things," she begins. "Brain chemistry plays a role, but it's only one piece of a much larger puzzle. Other causes can be a genetic predisposition, stressful or traumatic life events, illness, or gaslighting."

I look at her questioningly.

She uses an example I've told her from my childhood: "If you feel an emotion – for example fear, worry, or anxiety – and the person you confide in tells you that you're overreacting, you're just being dramatic and there is nothing to worry about, they invalidate your emotion. They're telling you that your emotion is wrong, which teaches you that you can't trust yourself. Over time, this creates a disconnect in yourself. If you can't trust yourself, you lose confidence, and you not only grow anxious about the world, but also about yourself. Teaching a child not to listen to their intuition does great damage that affects everything: their choice in career, what partner they end up with, how they perceive the world. It also makes them vulnerable to domineering partners, because if you don't trust yourself you're looking for someone you can trust, and predatory people can smell that. What may look like safety and caring can actually turn out to be an abusive relationship of dominance and control. But even if there were warning signs, you disregarded them, because you've learnt not to trust your gut feeling."

I stare at her, enthralled. "Oh my God, you are blowing my mind right now. This makes so much sense! I know exactly what you mean!"

I think back to my ill-fated brief relationship with Oliver in my early twenties, which I entered into despite having misgivings. I did it because my parents liked him so much and I was desperate to please them after the turbulent teenage years where we didn't get along.

I remember how I wanted to study journalism but gave up on the idea after being told that I wasn't smart or tough enough. A flood of memories is hitting me of times when I was super-excited about something, but at the smallest sign of doubt or discouragement from someone else I'd get deflated right away, believing them that my idea was stupid and that I couldn't do it.

"You can't make money with writing."

"Don't be so over-sensitive, you're such a drama queen."

"True love doesn't exist, look for someone who's compatible."

"Don't aim too high, you'll just end up disappointed."

"Why would anybody care to read about your *life?"*

Lola continues: "Consider something else: what do you think growing up in a society where you are objectified and shamed for it, treated like the lesser gender, taught to please and be nice and laugh about insults and not speak up does to you?" She pauses to let that sink in.

"Women have been gaslit for thousands of years. And when we speak up we're being labelled aggressive, hysterical, irrational, or asked if we're having our period. It collectively affects women's mental health, no matter if you're aware of it or not, and also creates generational trauma that's being passed on from one generation to the next."

I have never considered any of this. Feminism has always struck me as angry women hating all men, and I felt a bit sorry for them. In my world we used the word feminist as an insult, and I associated it with being unattractive, angry, and deeply unappealing. It speaks volumes that anger was a negative emotion for me, and that it was very important to me to be seen as both attractive and appealing. I fell for it all: the need to please, believing that I should be understanding and accommodating because "boys will be boys", that laughing about sexist jokes was a sign that I was open-minded and uncomplicated, that it was perfectly normal that more men than women were in positions of power, and that women who acted like men (being authoritative, confident, and not so fucking eager to please all the time) were cold-hearted bitches without a sense of humour.

Without being aware of it I had accepted that women were inferior to men, but at the same time I had also swallowed the lie that we are equal to men now, and that misogyny was a thing of the past. That disconnect messes with your brain because both can't be true at the same time. It's classic gaslighting, and until you recognize it you will question your own perception and sanity.

Lola lightly pokes at a spot in me that I've been noticing for a while but didn't dare touch. Did I really need any more turmoil in my life? Shouldn't I leave well enough alone? How would it affect my marriage if I started questioning the status quo? And what about my lifelong belief that I got along better with men than women, and that most women were bitches?

Each session I have with Lola digs deeper into long held beliefs by pulling them out of the deep, dark recesses of my mind into the light to examine them. And what I discover in the light of day and under her skillful guidance is that I've been living in a limited world with a bunch of made-up rules that I don't need to follow. All that shit that women are taught isn't a law that needs to be obeyed. Women don't need to see each other as rivals, it's something that the patriarchy benefits from and that keeps us at a disadvantage. The old boys club exists for a reason: men have helped each other succeed for millennia, creating the white men's world we all live in. Meanwhile, my own mother taught me not to trust other women, planting the seed that women were difficult and deceitful.

Despite years of actively unlearning stuff I was taught growing up, this one has proven to be almost impossible to shake. But awareness is the first step towards healing and working with Lola has the double-benefit of not only learning all this amazing information, but also seeing the proof right in front of me every time we connect.

The connection Lola and I have is one I want to cultivate with other women in my life: one of support, encouragement, warmth and laughter.

The biggest difference between therapy now as compared to therapy with Tori is that I'm not dreading my sessions with Lola. On the contrary, I'm starting to look forward to them, which is a new experience for me. I'm learning so much new stuff and new ways of thinking, it's fascinating!

Another huge difference is that I'm digging much deeper this time around. In the beginning of my therapy journey I only skimmed the surface of my problems. This was partly due to Tori and me not being as well suited to each other, but the other, bigger reason is that I've spent so many years pretending and hiding and not dealing with stuff that I actually don't know how to do it.

I don't even know *what* my problems are, only that I'm falling apart without knowing why.

That's the evil power of mental illness: it makes you doubt yourself, question your sanity, and tries to convince you that you're ungrateful and selfish. *You have no reason to feel down, just look at your life* she will whisper into your ear. *Loving husband, well-paying job, physical health, financial stability. You are better off than 99% of the world's population* (my depression likes statistics) *and you're still not happy? You are a spoiled, terrible human being. You should be ashamed of yourself.*

Lola helps me to unpack all of this. She teaches me the difference between shame-based self-attack and compassionate self-correction (the first one focuses on the past with the goal of punishment and shame; the second one focuses on growth, improvement, and hope for success), and she regularly reminds me that I *can* trust my intuition. "You know what's right for you," she keeps telling me, and that affirmation means the world to me. I didn't know how disconnected I felt from myself all these years until I'm starting to connect with my inner self.

But despite all the progress I'm making, there is one thing I haven't been able to talk about yet: my drinking. I like Lola so much that I can't imagine telling her the truth. It's such a weakness and so embarrassing, and I don't want her to think less of me. Somewhere inside me I know that she wouldn't judge me, that it's literally her job to be non-judgmental and to guide her clients through stuff like that, but I simply can't bring myself to confess. Half the time I'm able to tell myself that my drinking is normal, and the other half I do my best to avoid thinking about it. Pro tip: drinking is a *great* tactic to avoid thinking about drinking.

One morning I wake up with the fuzzy head I'm unfortunately well accustomed to. As I'm lying in bed, hungover and feeling terrible, I'm going through my routine checklist: what day is it? Wednesday. Am I working today? No, hence the hangover. What happened last night? Pause. Hm, that's odd – I can't seem to remember. *Shit.* That hasn't happened in a while, because I swore to myself after the last time that I would never let it get that far ever again. I tentatively turn to my husband and kiss him good morning.

"Morning babe," he mumbles. And then, after a moment: "You passed out in the bathroom last night." I freeze. Did I? I rack my brain, and sure enough, a blurry memory reluctantly swims to the surface: a tiled floor. Me curled up on it (after puking in the toilet? Can't remember.) And then – nothing. I have no recollection of how I got into bed. I can't remember what I did prior to ending up on the bathroom floor.

This is bad. The shame washes over me hot and sticky. I can feel the heat in my face, hot tears pricking my eyes. I've never felt so ashamed in my life. I want to die. Seriously, in this moment I want to die. How did I end up here? How is this happening to me? I'm frozen to the spot, wishing with all my heart that this is a bad dream and that I'm going to wake up any minute. This doesn't feel real; how can this be my life?

I slink out of bed quietly, not wanting to wake Richard who mercifully fell back asleep. As I'm standing in the kitchen, waiting for my coffee to finish brewing, I'm thinking back to last night.

It was a regular Tuesday night, nothing out of the ordinary. As soon as I came home from work I poured myself a glass of wine. Richard and I had a drink together, catching up on our respective days, and then he went outside to do chores. And what did I do? I sat down in front of my computer to "write", getting up regularly to refill my glass. I have no idea how many glasses I had.

That's the problem with boxed wine (and the reason why I buy it) – it's impossible to accurately know how much you're consuming in one sitting. Judging by my memory loss (I refuse to call it a blackout, even to myself) I'd say I drank the equivalent to two bottles. Looking around I surmise that I didn't cook dinner; a bottle and a half did it then.

Needless to say that I didn't do any actual writing. Even though the details are fuzzy, I can piece together how the evening went based on previous experience and flashes of memory: after staring at the screen for a while, unsuccessfully trying to work on my novel, I opened up YouTube to find some tunes for "inspiration". Before I knew it, two hours had passed in a blur of Avril Lavigne and Taylor Swift videos and going down the rabbit hole of botched celebrity plastic surgeries. After that? No idea, but at some point I ended up on the bathroom floor.

I bury my face in my hands and quietly cry for a while. I have therapy with Lola in a couple of hours, and I think this time I'll have to tell her. This is bad, and I clearly can't solve this problem on my own. I'm feeling nauseous just thinking about it, but there's a small part in me that feels desperate to share this terrible secret with someone who can help.

I take a shower and rehearse what I'm going to say to her.

"Lola, I'm drinking too much."

"I'm afraid I'm turning into an alcoholic."

"I blacked out last night."

"My drinking is out of control."

"Lola, I've been lying to do all this time about being on a mindfulness journey, I like drinking much better than meditating."

"On a scale from boring to just having a good time, how bad is waking up on the bathroom floor and not remembering how you got there? Oh, and did I mention that it happened on a regular Tuesday night, not after a wild party?"

Fuck, none of these are right. I'm getting more and more nervous, and I have no clue what to say. All the coffee isn't helping either, making me more jittery than I already am.

Ten minutes before my appointment I grab my phone, a glass of water and a roll of toilet paper (we're out of tissues) and head to my cabin. I have a She Shed next to our house that's my pride and joy, and it's supposed to serve as my sanctuary and sacred writing space. Ironically it morphed into our party space instead, and we've done quite a bit of drinking and celebrating in there. Will today be the day where the party ends?

I settle down at my desk and look at all the personal mementos I've collected over the years: the picture my sister painted of me with the caption "Let's write a new book"; the covers of the two books I've written; the little framed quote I put there for motivation that says "Don't give up! Someday, you'll be someone's favourite writer."

There's a little stone turtle that a Mexican street vendor gave me when I bought a wooden mask from him on vacation, a DIY candle holder one of the kids gave me for Christmas over fifteen years ago, and a homemade birthday card another one of the kids made me for my 40th birthday where she painted a corgi being lifted into the air by pink balloons.

I have such a wonderful life with so much love and support. I have a creative hobby I adore, all the dogs I ever wanted, a sanctuary filled with homemade gifts from friends and family. Why am I drinking? What am I running away from? Yes, I have this mental illness that kicks my ass sometimes, but aren't there so many great things that make more than up for it? Am I willing to risk losing it all for a few short hours of forgetting?

You can do this I tell myself when the screen comes to life and Lola's smiling face appears. *Go on, tell her.*

I don't tell her. All my courage falls out of my body the moment I open my mouth to speak, and what comes out is a complete surprise to me: I start babbling about my changing body and society's unrealistic expectation of women's bodies. What the fuck? If there's one aspect of growing up I've mastered it's my relationship to my body. After the typical body woes almost every woman goes through thanks to being taught that skinny is best and all that nonsense, I've made peace with my body years ago. I have 99 problems, but my body image isn't one of them, yet that's what I end up talking about during today's session.

Afterwards I slump in the chair, too disappointed in myself to get up. I missed my chance to ask Lola for help. If I didn't do it today, with the events from last night so fresh in my mind that I can practically still feel the tile imprinted on my body, I probably won't ever do it. Already I notice my brain kicking into self-defense mode, justifying, down-playing, rationalizing.

"What's done is done," "it can happen to anyone", "I didn't eat anything, that's why it happened", "it's been a stressful time".

In a few minutes I will go back to the house, crawl into bed with Richard and promise him that I'll never do it again. He will hug me tight and not give me a hard time about it; he never does. We will change the subject and go on with our day like nothing happened. I won't drink tonight.

By tomorrow I will have pushed the memory down into the pit where all the other unresolved problems are buried; and every time they threaten to come to the surface, guess what I will do?

Drink the medicine that helps me forget.

What a disaster. Am I going to live like this forever?

Flood

It happens just as predicted: I move on. With each passing day the memory fades a bit more, and I can almost pretend that it wasn't a big deal. If it weren't for my 2am-wakeups, everything would be dandy, but those damn middle-of-the-night scare-fests keep the humiliation alive. Still, time keeps on passing, and with no further incidents I'm doing a halfway decent job of convincing myself that my drinking is normal, and that life is finally returning to some semblance of normalcy.

And then something happens that makes everything else pale in comparison.

November has arrived, and with it unusually heavy rain. After the extremely dry summer with raging fires all around us the rain feels like a blessing, and it's extremely comfortable and cozy in our house with the fake fire on, candles burning, the dogs stretched out all over the place, and *Yellowstone* playing on the TV. We're both big fans, and one weekend we're starting the series over and spend all weekend watching John, Beth, Rip, and the rest of the gang riding horses, taking people that annoy them to the train station, defending their land, drinking like fish and looking hot doing it. Feeling rebellious, I even turn my phone off to be fully present in the moment, something I *never* do. My phone is usually permanently glued to my hand, but I feel the sudden urge for a little digital detox. It's a very pleasant weekend, and I wake up on Monday morning feeling well rested and refreshed.

It's still raining. Today I'm working my regular job 100 kilometres away, and the road I take, Highway 8, runs parallel to the Nicola River. As I'm driving alongside it I get the sense that the river is much higher than usual.

It's only 7am and still dark, but I catch glimpses of foaming waves, looking black in the darkness, and when I roll down my window a few inches I hear a roaring that I haven't heard here before. *That's weird*, I think to myself. The only time the river rises this much is in the spring after the snow melt, and only when we had a particularly snowy winter, which doesn't happen very often.

A few minutes into my drive I pass a section where water is lapping onto the road. I'm past it in seconds, and it's over so quickly that it takes a moment to sink in. *Wow, that was crazy,* I think, but the rest of the drive is uneventful. I'm leaving the river behind before it's light, and with the heavy rain it's difficult to see anything, so I'm unaware of how bad it is.

"What are you doing here?" That's how I'm greeted an hour later by the patient ambassador when I walk into work.

"I work here," I laugh, wondering if I got my days mixed up. Am I not supposed to be here today?

"Are you okay?" Taylor, the front desk clerk, rushes out of the office and looks at me with concern.

"Of course I am!" I answer bewildered. "Shouldn't I be?"

Now they're all looking at me as if I'm the one who's lost her mind, not them.

"What's going on?"

Understanding dawns on Taylor's face. "You really don't know, do you," she states.

"Know what?" I'm getting impatient. "What are you guys talking about?"

Taylor pulls me into her office. "Merritt is flooded," she tells me. "Part of the city has been evacuated."

"*What?!*" I can't believe it. "Are you sure?"

"Yes I'm sure, look." She opens up Facebook on her computer and shows me. Sure enough, there's a photo taken from one of the hills surrounding the city, showing Merritt submerged in water.

"Oh my God, that's insane." I explain: "I've been off my phone yesterday, and where we are there is nothing." I feel like the biggest idiot for not knowing that this is happening. I look again at the grainy image taken at dawn, with water filling up every road like a macabre parody of Venice, Italy.

"I'm glad you're okay," Taylor says to me. "I was worried."

"We live up on a hill, we are fine," I assure her. "The Nicola was pretty high this morning, but it could never reach us. We are hundreds of feet above it. I just hope everybody living close to it is okay."

I head to my desk and fire up the computer right away to catch up on this insane turn of events. We live in the semi-desert – how can we be flooded?

But sure enough, more images keep popping up. With the increasing daylight they become clearer, and I'm still staring at the latest picture that shows muddy brown water covering every surface of the city when the latest comes in: the entire city is being evacuated. I jump up and run to the front office. "Merritt is being evacuated!" I yell. "I'm going home, in case they're closing the roads." We are not included in the evacuation order, but I still have vivid memories of just a few short months ago when one road after another was being shut down, and there have been reports of road closures due to mud slides and flooding. I grab my stuff and rush to my car shortly after 11 am. Without thinking, I turn onto the familiar road home – Highway 8.

It's only been four hours since I drove past it earlier this morning, but boy oh boy, a lot has changed. The river is *raging*. It looks like boiling water, foaming angrily, its edge licking hungrily at the bridge I'm driving over. The water is almost level with the road, and it has started to flood it in several places. It's still raining hard and I'm feeling distinctly uneasy, but I keep driving because I have only one goal in my mind: to make it home as fast as possible. The highway is lowest in the section I'm currently on before rising higher above river level, and I figure if I make it through the next ten or so kilometers I will be fine.

But then I drive around a bend, and what I see makes me want to vomit. *THERE'S A PIECE OF THE ROAD MISSING.* A big, triangular-shaped piece of pavement has broken off, gone along with the guardrail that's also missing. But instead of stopping and reassessing (or turning around and getting the hell outta there), my right foot seems to be glued to the gas pedal. I simply steer over to the left side and keep on driving, squeezing myself as close to the rock face as possible to avoid the gaping hole, noticing as I'm crawling past it that there's a large crack in my half of the road that I'm currently driving over. Only when I'm past that insanely unsafe section do I finally stop the car. Heart pounding I get out to take a closer look, and that's when the fear sets in. "*Holy shit*", I say under my breath. Did I really just drive on a crumbling road that's falling apart beneath my tires? I snap a couple quick pictures and then I jump back into the car, eager to get away as quickly as possible. There's no explanation why I keep going when I have to assume that there are worse parts ahead of me that must be flooded by now. I'm on autopilot since my brain has stopped working, and my autopilot clearly isn't very smart. I'm also in denial about the severity of the situation because it's just so unlikely. Stuff like this doesn't happen in real life, right? Despite the evidence to the contrary I'm clinging on to the notion that this must have been the worst of it because everything else just doesn't make sense.

Think again, sister. Not even five minutes later I encounter something just as unlikely as the giant hole. In front of me is water. The surging river is lapping in big waves onto the highway, which is covered in brown, foaming water. The river also deposited a large amount of driftwood onto the road, and that's what's really making me stop and assess my situation. If not for the obstacle blocking my way I would just keep on going and plow through the water, but the driftwood makes that impossible. I'm seriously considering the feasibility of trying to clear the wood away, when luckily a truck pulls up on the other side of the flooded road. It belongs to a highway employee, and he yells at me to turn around and get out while I still can, making shooing motions with his arms when I don't react right away.

Grateful that someone is telling me what to do, I turn around. And that's when it dawns on me that I will have to cross the half-ripped-off part of the road again. Even though I nonchalantly drove over it only minutes earlier like it's no big deal, now I have vivid visions of tumbling down into the raging waters, never to surface again. I'm freaking out, so I call Richard.

"I have to drive back over the broken-off bit, and I'm scared!!" I wail, with no need to elaborate because I've kept him up to date on my progress thoroughly throughout the drive.

"Can you stay with me until I'm past it?" I beg, and he agrees.

"It's coming up!" I yell.

"Nope, not yet, sorry," a moment later.

"I'll stay with you the entire time," he promises calmly.

A minute later, I really do see the ominous crack in the road ahead of me. Did it get bigger? I think it did. It certainly seems about 100 times scarier than it did just a little while ago.

I take a deep breath, and then squeeze my car as close to the rock face as I can. My passenger side mirror is scraping the side of the wall, which tells me that this is as far as I can go to the side.

The only way I have left now is straight through.

"I'm going across it now!" I yell at Richard, and then, with both hands gripping the steering wheel in a death grip, I drive across.

"Aaaaaahhhhhhhh!!" I scream, and then it's over.

I'm on the other side, and with tears streaming down my face, I drive on, shaking violently.

"Are you okay? Did you make it?" Richard shouts, not knowing what happened. The last thing he heard was my scream. I nod numbly, before realizing that he can't see me.

"Yes, I am. I'm safe," I say.

It takes me over two hours to get home, and when I sink into Richard's arms I start crying again. "I was terrified," I sob into his shoulder, and he hugs me tightly, relieved that I made it home safely.

Over the next few days we learn the extent of the damage, and it's shocking. Highway 8 is destroyed in eighteen sections, meaning that it's completely gone in those places. Where there once was a road there is now nothing. I get chills watching the helicopter footage, realizing how close I came to endangering my life.

But that's not the worst of it. I watch in horror on the news as someone's house gets swept away by the raging water. It literally falls into the river and gets carried away – *an entire house*. I wouldn't believe it was possible, but there is the shaky footage of a house gone within seconds. I drove past that place every day on my way to work, know the owner, know where he works.

He went within minutes from homeowner to literally being home-less, all his worldly possessions gone.

Merritt is unrecognizable. The entire town of over 7,000 people has been evacuated, the drinking water is contaminated, and the sewage system is not working due to the city's wastewater treatment plant being flooded.

Hours after the official evacuation order the city erects barricades at every entry point to prevent people from entering. Access to Merritt is officially prohibited. Some people have decided to stay behind, either because they have pets, no place to go, or because they're afraid of looting. With no drinking water or working toilet "it's like camping", one of them jokes. It started snowing on the day of the flood, which is handy because people can melt snow and boil it for drinking water.

The residents of the long-term care facilities and hospital patients need to be relocated, and once that's done the hospital closes. It will stay closed for nearly two weeks.

All major highways but one have been damaged, entire bridges are washed away, and mud slides have taken away roads, bridges – and people. Horrific stories surface of cars being engulfed by mud slides with people still inside them. Others were luckier but had to go through days of being stranded on the road, often without food or water in freezing temperatures. We hear about thousands of horses, cattle, chickens, and other livestock having drowned. Other animals will have to be put down in the following days due to hypothermia.

Merritt isn't the only community that has been severely hit. Several other towns are equally badly affected, even though none of them need to be completely evacuated, and nobody knows if the danger is over. There are rumours of more atmospheric rivers possibly hitting us, but thankfully they turn out not to be true.

What is an *atmospheric river* you may wonder? That's the event that caused the mess we are in. Simply put, it's "a large, narrow stream of water vapour that travels through the sky".[10]

That water vapour, sometimes referred to as "rivers in the sky" can "stretch to 1,600 kilometres long and more than 640 kilometres wide, and on average, carries an amount of water equivalent to 25 Mississippi Rivers", according to Marty Ralph, a researcher and director at the University of California San Diego's Scripps Institution of Oceanography. That massive amount of water can be dropped over large areas in a short amount of time, like turning on the shower at full blast and letting it rip for a while.

On the weekend preceding November 15, the day of the flood, several things happened that created the perfect storm. There was record-breaking rainfall thanks to the atmospheric river across large areas of Western British Columbia. Furthermore, the warm rain melted snow in the mountains that added extra water to the deluge. And to top it off, there was the damage from the forest fires. Not only does a lack of trees make landslides much more common, but the soil in forested areas can turn hydrophobic after severe fires, meaning the soil's particles repel water due to waxy compounds that are being distributed across the forest floor after wildfires.[11] That water repellence makes absorption of water much more difficult, resulting in runoffs.

Thanks to this series of unfortunate events we are now in yet another state of emergency. They keep coming hard and fast in 2021, aren't they? I think this is number three in our province, but I could be wrong. I've lost count at this point with all the catastrophes happening all the time.

Vancouver is cut off by land from the rest of Canada, but I don't have any energy left in me to care. The politicians yammer on about how the highway closures impact the "transport networks and movement of essential goods and supplies", but I don't pay much attention. We've been permanently in a state of heightened tension for almost two years, and my tank is empty. Besides, I have more pressing things to worry about.

---

[10] CBC, What are atmospheric rivers, and how are the affecting the B.C. floods?, https://www.cbc.ca/radio/whatonearth/what-are-atmospheric-rivers-and-how-are-they-affecting-the-b-c-floods-1.6253763

[11] Wikipedia, Hydrophobic soil, https://en.wikipedia.org/wiki/Hydrophobic_soil

With my beloved highway out of commission for the foreseeable future, I have to take the only other route left: Highway 97C. I call it the high road because it's approximately 800m/2,624f higher than my usual route, and first you climb, climb, climb up the mountain only to then drive down a very steep, very long hill on the other side. I've never driven it in the winter because it has the reputation of being one of the worst roads around, but now I have no choice.

On the very next day after the flood I head to this new-to-me-in-the-winter highway towards work.

Remember how I mentioned that it started snowing the day of the flood? Merritt, with an elevation of 605m got little more than a light dusting.

Highway 97C is more than twice as high, and the weather is completely different up there. As I'm going up higher and higher I see to my dismay that it doesn't just live up to its reputation of being awful in the winter – it exceeds it by a mile.

The road has completely disappeared. All I can see is a long stretch of white, indistinguishable from the surrounding landscape. There's not a sliver of blacktop peeping through the snow, and the only reason I can make out where the road is hiding is by the glossy tire tracks that have been left by other vehicles and that are shining like glass in the morning sunshine, warning me of their slipperiness. I carefully drive in the middle of the road, keeping an eye on the rear-view mirror for other cars that might be approaching from behind. But no other cars are coming – I seem to be the only one out in this snowscape.

What unsettles me is that there is no guardrail on this highway. In several areas it sits high on a ridge, with nothing between me and several hundred feet of steep slope that lead to the bottom of the embankment on either side. All I need is one second of losing control of my car and I could end up falling off the mountain. Even if it doesn't kill me right away, there is no cell service, and it's very likely that nobody would see me from the road. Could I die a long and painful death on this stupid highway?

I usually don't get nervous while driving, but this road scares me. I'm white knuckling it all the way to work, bathed in sweat, and when I finally turn off the engine I sit there, dazed. Houston, we have a problem. I have six months of winter driving ahead of me and I have no idea if I'll be able to do it. I'm a nervous wreck. Predictions for Highway 8 are that it will be closed for one to two *years*.

What am I gonna do now?

And Just Like That

The fog is thick and dense. It's still dark outside, and with the impenetrable fog I can see nothing but a white wall surrounding me. Visibility? What visibility? I'm crawling at a speed of less than 50km/h, hoping the fog will clear at some point. Even though I've left two hours early, I may be late if I have to drive the entire 100 kilometers at this snail's pace.

BAM!

I hit the brakes, remembering at the last split second not to slam them down too hard in case of ice. A deer jumped right in front of my car, literally out of nowhere. I didn't hit it. Before I have time to breathe a sigh of relief, I catch movement to my left out of the corner of my eye – another deer. Its head pops up like an apparition in my side window, then it's gone again. I keep driving on autopilot, trying to process what just happened: did a deer almost run into my car – right after I almost hit *another* deer? What the hell?!

It takes a while for my wildly beating heart to calm down. As I am winding my way up the mountain I leave the fog behind, rising above it like a phoenix out of the ashes into the rising sun. It's mesmerizing. I see more deer along the way, but fortunately none of them are on the road.

It's been two weeks since the day of the flood. To my utter disbelief, I've gotten used to the drive. Well, "gotten used to" may be overstating it – I've resigned myself to the fact that I have no other option. Quitting my job seemed too extreme a reaction, but don't think that I didn't consider it. Instead of quitting I bought myself studded winter tires for the first time, because it helps with driving on ice, which seems to be a permanent fixture up there.

I miss Highway 8 desperately. I fondly think back to the mama bear with her cub I saw just a few weeks ago, and I hope that the horses and the wild sheep are okay. Most of the horses aren't wild, they have owners who let them roam free during the summer and feed hay in the winter, but everybody who lives there has been evacuated. Will the horses survive the winter?

The familiar heaviness is descending upon me again. It's like a wet blanket that settles itself over me, blocking the light and threatening to suffocate me. Tears are pricking my eyes when I see the "Welcome back Health Care Team" sign in front of the hospital and I almost start bawling at the sight of the handwritten "Welcome back" scrawled on a piece of white water and taped to the door of Walmart.

I do start crying during the Santa parade and leave at once to avoid concerned questions from other spectators. What would I tell them if they asked me if something's wrong?

"Nothing to worry about dear, it's just my depression. Carry on!" For a wild moment I wish I would try it just to see the reaction, but I know I can't. I'm at my weakest and most vulnerable when I enter a depression. I feel ashamed and small, and my flight instinct is overpowering, compelling me to run away and hide.

I crawl into bed five minutes later, hoping desperately that I won't get called to the hospital. I wish for nothing more than to be able to turn off my phone and shut the world out for a while and having to be "on" feels like a superhuman effort I don't have the energy for.

There's an analogy that I've been using for years that explains that particular tiredness. It's called the "Spoon Theory", and it was created by Christine Miserandino, a writer and speaker who lives with lupus, a chronic autoimmune disease. Lupus is one of the diseases that's sometimes referred to as invisible because you can't tell by looking at someone that they have it. When Christine's friend asks her one day over coffee what it feels like to live with a chronic disease, Christine comes up with the spoon theory. She grabs a bunch of spoons and explains to her friend that the spoons represent energy, and how someone with a chronic disease has a limited number of spoons as opposed to someone who's healthy.

I find that the spoon theory also applies to the exhaustion that comes with a depressive episode, because my energy reserves are limited during that time as well.

You don't realize how many steps there are involved in a callback until your spoons are limited:

1. Phone rings. I have to pick up and talk to whoever is calling = one spoon. (I find phones stressful and would let it go to voice mail if I could. Since I can't it drains some of my energy.)
2. Get out of bed, run brush through rats' nest that's hair, brush teeth if I haven't done it yet that day (which I won't have on a depressed day) = one spoon.
3. Get dressed, make sure I have hospital keys and phone, put on coat and shoes, try to unlock car and realize I forgot car keys, walk back into house to search for car keys, can't find them because my brain doesn't function properly, finally find them tangled up in the covers of my bed, all the while starting to panic because I'm wasting so much time and I should get going because we have to be at the hospital within a certain period of time = two spoons.
4. The drive, arrival, turning on of machine and computer, checking the order, setting up of the x-ray room, taking a deep breath to mentally prepare to deal with a patient who may be seriously injured or confused or angry or scared takes another spoon.
5. Now I'm heading to the ER to get the patient. I stick my head into the nurse's station to say hi and check if there's anything I need to know, and once they've brought me up to speed I go to collect the patient. The thing about working in emergency is that you never know what walks through the door. It could be someone who is intoxicated, mentally ill, suicidal, bleeding profusely, someone with dementia or an anti-masker who's taken offense to the mask mandate in the hospital. It may also be someone who's very nice and appreciative of me coming in for their x-ray, or it could be someone who will receive the worst news of their

lives thanks to the images I'm about to take. The uncertainty is what keeps it interesting on good days, but on bad ones it's draining and can cost another few spoons.
6. Depending on the exam ordered, the level of cooperation of the patient, the injury and how well my brain is functioning the exam can go anywhere from 1 (easy) to 10 (need to call a code/security/help because the patient has a cardiac arrest/gets aggressive/collapses). Therefore, the number of spoons required varies wildly according to the situation at hand.
7. Sometimes there are x-rays ordered on more than one patient, so I'm repeating the previous steps. Other times I'm done, and once the patient has been returned to the ER and I have completed the paperwork, shut down the department and said bye to the nurses I go home and collapse on my bed.

Steps 1-7 may be repeated up to twelve times on a weekend (my record of call backs thus far). That's a *lot* of spoons you're using up when you're having a series of bad mental health days. And what happens when you've run out of spoons? Then it's game over. It's like a car that ran out of gas – once it's empty it's not going anywhere. But since I know that I need to keep a few spoons on hand because I'm on call and *have* to function, I need to be extremely careful with my limited energy. Anything that drains it needs to be avoided at all costs, which for me means no small talk, not looking at the news, no human interaction unless absolutely necessary (if I don't reply to your text, that's why), ideally no social media, and sometimes no shower or decent food. Instead I sleep lots, or if I can't sleep I watch something easy on Netflix, maybe read, and on not-too-bad days I might even go for a walk. But walking is usually out when I'm in a depression because I'm too tired for any physical exertion.

It's December, and December has always been a bad month for me. Not only do I have mixed feelings about the whole Christmas craziness (some years I like parts of it, others I hate it all), but it's also the month of my birthday, and mixed feelings doesn't even begin to describe how I feel about my birthday.

It's not that I have a problem with getting older – quite the opposite. I *love* getting older, because being young is immensely stressful. So much pressure about the way you look, about having kids, about finding the right partner and the right career and cultivating a group of friends. You have to figure out taxes and what you like in bed, choose who you want to vote for, and decide if you're going to be a woman who wears lipstick or colourless lip balm. You have no idea what makes you happy and all of life seems to be an endless exercise in trial and error. *So* much error.

Being young is exhausting and extremely overrated.

The problem with my birthday is that I never know how to celebrate it. One part of me wants a party, ideally a party completely planned and executed by someone else where I have to do nothing but show up. I imagine lots of glitter and balloons, happy people in stylish outfits, beautifully wrapped presents, a big birthday cake and most important of all, the right attitude to enjoy it all and not cringe at being the centre of attention.

However, this expectation is flawed because a) I don't have the kind of spouse who could pull any of it off, and b) I'm usually in a depression in December.

Option c) is throwing it myself, but thanks to my seasonal depression I usually don't do it. Besides, it's Christmas season, and if you want to have a birthday party you're competing against Christmas parties, cookie exchanges, gingerbread decorating competitions and a ton of other Christmas-related events.

That's a lot of pressure, which explains why the number of parties I've organized for myself is less than a handful in 25 years. Most of the time I buy a couple of bottles of champagne, bake myself a cake and just stay at home with my husband, eating cake and drinking champagne. Some years I'm enjoying myself, since it's an introvert's dream and I love staying home, but if it's a depression-birthday the champagne backfires and makes me feel weepy, unloved and like a loser. I still always drink it though because it's a birthday tradition.

This year, in a moment that I can only attribute to temporary insanity, I decide it's about time to have myself a little birthday party. The desire is born out of a combination of being fed up with feeling down, having survived all the catastrophes this year, and wanting an occasion to get dressed up for. I also like to pretend once in a while that I'm completely normal, and I've actually planned and hosted quite a few great parties over the years – just usually not for me. Richard's birthday is in June, and we've celebrated his birthday at a ratio of approximately 4:1 in comparison to mine.

The major highways are still closed after the flood, which means I can't invite friends who live out of town. That suits me fine, because I seem to be more nervous than I remember being in the past and want to keep the party small.

At the day of the party I get up extra early to prepare everything. I'm doing a Christmas-themed buffet with a candy-shaped Caprese platter, a Christmas-tree cheese ball, Christmas-tree shaped pizzas, and a couple of different salads and nibbles. At lunch time I have my first glass of wine to calm my nerves because I'm anxious. I've had all of our friends over lots of times, and I'm usually never nervous around any of them. Is it because I haven't hosted a party in two years? Have I gotten rusty? Where is this annoying anxiety coming from?

With everything ready and over two hours to go before anyone arrives I decide to take a bath. I pour myself another glass of wine and sink slowly into the warm water, trying to relax. But my mind is spinning, going over everything that could go wrong: nobody is coming, the food tastes terrible, everybody is bored or having an awful time. I try to stop the tidal wave of bad thoughts by turning it around and telling myself all the things that could go right, but my brain isn't having it. It wants to catastrophize, and it won't be distracted from that goal by a little bit of positive thinking. Since I can't relax I declare defeat, shave my legs, wash my hair, and then climb out of the bath after barely fifteen minutes, which is like five seconds in bath-time.

I top up my glass (how did it get empty so fast?) and start getting ready. At this point I'm torn between the urge to cancel everything and wanting people to arrive **now** so my pre-guest anxiety can get lost. I'm regretting organizing this whole party-thing, because right now nothing sounds better than curling up on the couch with my dogs and looking dreamily at my Christmas tree without anybody else there. But it's too late for that now, and the only way out of this is through.

"Thank God for alcohol," I mutter to myself, and proceed to use those words as my guiding principle for the evening.

Everybody shows up. They bring cards and gifts and good cheer. They all enjoy the food, evidenced by the fact that they eat a lot of it, which is the biggest compliment a cook can get. We laugh and talk and have a good time. I wear my red dress and gold sparkly shoes, soon to be kicked off. My hair is curled, and I've put some mascara on.

When everybody is fed and happy we settle into the living room, the soft glow of the Christmas tree making the room look magical. I'm relaxed now, flushed from several glasses of wine and relieved that the hard part is over. This is easy; this is fun.

My recollection from the rest of the night is blurry. We laugh; we drink some more; we talk about I don't know what. After a few hours our guests leave with hugs goodbye. Once everybody is gone I fall onto the couch, exhausted but pleased.

"That was a great party, don't you think?" I ask Richard.

"It was wonderful. Well done babe," he agrees.

"I didn't take any pictures!" I suddenly remember. "Let's do a selfie!"

I jump up, hug him from behind and snap a picture of us. We are both smiling and looking happy. It's the last clear memory I have.

The rest is stored in my head as jagged, disconnected pieces: me shouting. Richard grumbling. Me crying. The angry pour of yet another glass that neither of us needs. I'm yelling hurtful things; at some point he's yelling back. Eventually I stumble to bed, sobbing and distraught. I can't remember the reason because there is no reason. Or to be more specific, the reason is that I drank too much.

I fall into a restless sleep, only to be awakened a few hours later at 2am, my personal witching hour. I stare at the ceiling, the familiar self-loathing washing over me. I feel like death warmed over. Why do I keep doing this to myself? Why did I have to ruin a wonderful evening by drinking too much? I replay the night in my head, relieved to confirm that I didn't embarrass myself in front of our friends. No, I usually keep that special treat for me and my husband. I rarely get that drunk in front of others because I despise losing control in public. But what does that say about me that I care more about how others see me than I see myself? Am I not worthy of treating myself with the same respect?

A few days later I'm back in the staff residence for my weekend of call. Richard and I made up the day after the party, and even though everything has been fine between us I'm feeling uneasy. I can't shake off the fight and my behaviour. To distract myself I'm watching *And Just Like That...*, the sequel to *Sex and the City*.

I always have and always will love SATC. I adore the outfits and seeing NYC as the fifth heroine of the show. I'm a country girl who would hate living in any city, let alone one as noisy and chaotic as New York, but I can't get enough of seeing it on TV. SATC is one of my feel-good shows, it saw me through a major heartbreak in my early twenties, and it is great fun to watch. I'm thrilled that they made a new spin-off, and so far I'm loving it.

My friend Alex is also watching and loving the new series, and we keep texting each other as we watch. It's the episode where Charlotte finds the mini liquor bottles in Miranda's backpack, and when she tries to talk to Carrie about it Carries brushes her off, saying dismissively that she wishes Charlotte would "stop noticing things".

Alex sends me a meme about it:

Charlotte: I think Miranda has a drinking problem.

Carrie: Can you shut the fuck up?

My response: *"Charlotte has always been the judgmental prissy one, she's my least favourite"*

My friend's reply: *"I feel like she's more worried than judgey about this in particular, but it'll depend on how she deals with it."*

That mild, innocent answer hits me like a bucket of ice-cold water. I recoil, and then I feel heat rise in my face. It feels as if a very bright, very hot spotlight has been turned on and is trained on me, pinning me in place like a dead butterfly on a board. I feel exposed and found out. *Is she talking about me?! Is she trying to tell me something?*

I throw my phone next to me on the couch, draw my knees into my chest and stare into space. My heart is racing, and I can feel adrenaline flooding my body. My body is reacting as if it's threatened and ready to flee at any moment.

I force myself to breathe slowly, deep breaths in and longer breaths out. I've read somewhere that exhaling longer than inhaling calms down the nervous system, and my nervous system needs calming down STAT, because it's currently firing on all cylinders.

The breathing helps. As I feel my heart slow down, I start to analyze the text exchange I've had with Alex. She's a good friend and we are in touch regularly, but I only see her two to three times a year. She's never seen me drunk. True, one time I called her in alcohol-fuelled desperation in the midst of a terrible depression that had pulled me down so deep that I thought I would never make it out. That was years ago though. She doesn't know how much I drink or how much it's been stressing me out. That physical reaction I just had? That's my body trying to tell me something.

Miranda is 55 in the show. I'm 42. If I continue the way I have been drinking, maybe slowly increasing the amount because I'll need more and more alcohol for the desired effect, where will I be when I'm 55? Will I have people talking behind my back, either out of concern or in a disbelieving "did you see what she did?"-kinda way?

Will I look as great as Miranda in the show does? Absolutely not. I regularly see heavily-drinking women in my line of work, and no amount of make-up or surgery can hide the effect of too much booze over too many years. Best case scenario, I will be bloated and flabby and tired, feeling uncomfortable in my saggy skin with dark circles under my bloodshot eyes.

Other possible scenarios: shaky hands, liver disease, breast cancer, pancreatitis, broken relationships, DUIs, worsening depression, increased anxiety, maybe some suicidal thoughts thrown in.

Worst case scenario: death.

Even without the scary mental and physical health implications, what will my life look like on a daily basis if I continue on the path I'm on?

I imagine myself in thirteen years. Still working the same job, heading straight to the fridge as soon as I come home to pour myself the first of several glasses of wine, flopping down on the sofa, thinking of all the things I want to do but postpone until tomorrow.. There are a *lot* of tomorrows between now and then, and as I'm sitting here, rooted to the spot by dread and that bright spotlight trained on me, I have an epiphany: I will achieve none of my goals if I don't make a radical change.

In thirteen long years I will have achieved nothing if I keep on doing what I've been doing. And I'm not talking about fame and fortune – I'm talking about personal growth, looking after my body, mind, and soul, becoming a woman I'm proud of. Do I still want to wake up with self-loathing several nights a week when I'm in my 50s? Will I still numb my feelings because I'm too scared to face them? Will I still "work on my book" in thirteen years from now, finding a million excuses why I haven't finished it, when the biggest reason is my wine habit? If the last two years, my heaviest drinking years, are a preview of things to come, the future is looking bleak. It's easy to blame the pandemic for everything, to point at the fires and the flood and the stress at work and the dismal state of the world and say, "poor me. Look at all the shit that's been happening to me. No wonder I haven't been able to write. Once all these problems are gone *then* I will be able to write again".

Pff, as if. The thing about problems is, they never end. And the thing about anxiety is that it causes your brain to overthink and catastrophize and make up a gazillion terrible scenarios. Even if the pandemic ends and there will never be forest fires or floods ever again, my brain will find other things to worry about. Which in turns translates to other reasons to drink about.

And if I've learnt anything over the last two years, it's this: I can't write when I drink the way I have. Writing is the thing that fills me up most in the world, that makes me feel most alive and accomplished – and I haven't been doing it. Because I've been too busy drinking.

I have a choice to make: wine or writing.

Shrinking or expanding.

Hiding or fighting.

Existing or *living*.

Grey Area Drinking

The Monday following that weekend is my first test. Usually that's a day where I always drink as reward for three days of no alcohol. Not today though; today is the first day of the rest of my life.

It's also a day off, which complicates things. Instead of having to face only an evening of resisting temptation I have an entire day ahead of me, and it is going to be a long one. The first thing I do is get rid of the white wine that's still in the fridge. I pour it down the drain, wondering if that was the last white wine I've ever bought in my life. That thought is unsettling, so I shove it down into the pit to join the other unresolved issues. There's more booze in the house, spirits and leftover red wine from the party, but those have never tempted me much, so I leave them in the cupboard. It gives me a much-needed feeling of accomplishment that I've never poured whatever alcohol there is available down my throat. Surely a sign that I'm not addicted? I can't imagine drinking vodka straight from the bottle, let alone mouthwash or hand sanitizer.

That done I still have a lot of day left before I can go to bed; it's only 9:30 in the morning.

What would I normally do? I ask myself. I've never started drinking in the morning – why does it suddenly seem so impossible to simply go about my day?

I do my best to distract myself. I go grocery-shopping, noticing for the first time the two different non-alcoholic wines tucked in next to the soft drinks, and grabbing a bottle just in case; dispose of our recycling; take Lily for a walk; cook dinner. It's now the middle of the afternoon with dusk approaching rapidly, and with it the danger zone. This is the time where I would normally pour myself a glass of wine. It's cold and dark outside, cozy and warm inside, and I miss wine with an intensity that's as powerful as it is scary. My wily brain is bombarding me with its familiar conviction tactics: *you deserve it; you just had three days of not drinking; life's too short to deprive yourself; you're fine, you never drink hard liquor; everybody drinks wine, it's just fermented grapes, totally natural and harmless.* That same voice that's currently trying to seduce me into drinking will turn on me a few hours down the road, berating me for my weakness and calling me a failure and a lush.

Grateful that I got rid of temptation this morning, I pour myself a glass of the non-alcoholic wine I bought.

It tastes terrible. Still, beggars can't be choosers, so I clutch it tightly in my hand and wander aimlessly through the house, trying to decide how to spend the next few hours before I can escape into bed. I flick through Netflix but can't decide what to watch. I consider taking a bath, but the thought of getting wet and my feet getting all wrinkly turns me off. (Yes, I've turned into a cranky toddler.) I flop down on my bed and scroll through Instagram, bored while I'm doing it, when an idea pops into my head. I type the word *sober* into the search bar and hold my breath. The first suggested page that pops up is called *Sober Celebrities* and I eagerly click on it. The more faces and names I see the wider my smile gets. Brad Pitt, Bradley Cooper, Jessica Simpson, Chrissy Teigen, Eminem, Gerard Butler, Florence Welch, Jamie Lee Curtis ... the list goes on and on. These people are *cool*! For the first time all day I feel excitement rather than dread about my future. Could it be that the fun doesn't stop once alcohol has left the building?

I hit the "Follow"-button, slightly concerned that someone may notice and wonder why I'm suddenly following a sober account. But then I remind myself that nobody cares whom I'm following, and besides, anything related to celebrities is irresistible to most. Even if someone should see and question my choice, I could always say that I'm simply curious about celebrities.

Then I stop and say out loud: "What is wrong with you? Stop overthinking this!"

The shame surrounding my drinking runs deep.

Shame is also the reason why I don't tell Richard right away that I've decided to quit/cut back (still not certain which one it will be), because he's heard that old chestnut a few too many times in the past only to see me return to my old ways shortly after. I want to make sure that this time it's different. It *feels* different, but I can't quite figure out why, and I decide I need to work out what the difference is before I share my decision with him.

It takes me a while before I can put my finger on it, but when I finally do I can't believe how obvious it is. But isn't that always the case? The most complicated questions have the simplest answers. And the difference is as simple as it is profound: every time before I didn't really *want* to quit drinking. I wanted to stop drinking so much and to return to the days when I truly was a moderate drinker who could take it or leave it. But quitting for good? I hadn't wanted that.

This time I do. I have reached the point where I know I've had enough, and where I stand at a crossroads. I could continue on the road I am on, or I could stop. There is no third option. I have spent years chasing the elusive "moderate drinking" option despite failing time and time again, like a dieter trying every new diet, convinced that *this* one will finally stick. Even though I don't know (yet) why I have failed to return to my former moderate drinking self that I've been for most of my life, I have finally come to realize that I will never be able to go back to it. Fiftieth time's the charm? It won't be.

As the weeks pass slowly (the days seem much longer now since I quit drinking), I read and re-read every quit lit book I can get my hands on. *This Naked Mind* by Annie Grace, *Dry* by Augusten Burroughs, *The Unexpected Joy of Being Sober* by Catherine Gray, *The Sober Lush* by Amanda Eyre Ward and Jardine Libaire, *Blackout: Remembering the Things I Drank to Forget* by Sarah Hepola, *Nothing Good Can Come from This* by Kristi Coulter.

Not only does it help tremendously to read about the experiences of other women (and Augusten) who have quit booze and/or drugs, I'm also finally finding an answer to a question that's plagued me forever:

Am I an alcoholic?

I've asked myself that question dozens of times over the years, terrified of the answer. I thought there were only two options: either you belonged into the category of people who could "drink responsibly", or you were an alcoholic. I desperately didn't want to end up in the latter, because that life didn't seem worth living: having to go to AA meetings in dusty church basements and telling a bunch of strangers for the rest of your life that you had an incurable disease you were powerless against, forever craving something you could no longer have? No thanks.

[Before I continue I want to emphasize that I don't mean to minimize AA's importance to many people's sobriety. I know that it has saved countless lives and continues to be a lifeline of hope for many. I have a complicated relationship with the church and religion, so it's not for me personally.]

If that wasn't an option, then logic dictated that I must be a "normal" drinker. To support this self-diagnosis I'd do those quizzes that tell you if you're drinking too much, and there is a way of doing them that will reassure you that you're perfectly fine: focus on the questions that make you feel good about yourself and ignore the rest. It works for right-wing politicians and pro-lifers, why shouldn't it work for you?

1. Do you drink daily?

Nope, I don't. Score! I've never been a daily drinker, so there. Shoutout to being on call for my job and to my anxiety who won't permit me to drink every single night due to overwhelming shame and self-loathing. Thanks, girl.

2. Do you drink in the morning?

No. I'm neither a Baileys-in-my-coffee nor a mimosa gal (I preferred my champagne undiluted), so I never started earlier than noon-ish.

3. Do you have alcohol withdrawal symptoms?

It never got that far. Phew! Did I regularly check my hands for any suspicious shaking or my skin-tone for a tinge of yellow? Yes I did. But I have a mental illness and I'm a chronic overthinker and catastrophizer, so you have to take my behaviour with a grain of salt.

4. Do you prioritize drinking over family, your job, or anything else in your life?

Have I skipped a hike and gone straight to post-hike drinks (which makes them just drinks, I guess)? Sure. Hasn't everyone?

But I've never called in sick to work because of drinking or a hangover, and I'm much more likely to skip social engagements due to my social anxiety and introvertism than flaking out because I want to drink.

I'd skip over the sections that mentioned the recommendation of not drinking more than one glass per day for women (surely nobody drank only *one* glass of wine?), *never* drinking more than four drinks in one day (these people clearly have never been to a German Oktoberfest), or the pesky question of "have you ever woken up and not remembered what happened the night before?" (The only honest answer to that question was "yes, several times" – which is why I usually avoided answering it.)

I'd also make sure to pay close attention to every article that said that wine was good for one's heart, and to remind myself that the Mediterranean diet was supposedly the healthiest diet in the world, and it included plenty of wine, didn't it?

Still, the nagging voices inside my head kept on nagging. Some say that if you have to ask yourself if you have a drinking problem, chances are you do.

As I immerse myself in sober literature and dip my toes into the sober community online, I discover a term that fits my situation much better than the outdated "alcoholic" (now replaced with "person with alcohol abuse disorder"): grey area drinker.

Grey area drinking is the undefined space between the moderate drinker and the dependent one – a wild land with no rules, with many more shades of grey than just 50. As soon as I hear of it I nod my head in recognition: of *course* this is the place I've inhabited all these years. The lack of hard and fast definitions and the ability to keep myself at the moderate drinking end by using the above method of test-taking, selective reading, and the right company (i.e. people who drink more than I do) appealed to me before I even knew that category existed.

Anything goes in the grey area: drinking every day for a year and then quitting for six months; using alcohol as treat, medicine, or reward, and withholding it as punishment; playing the delightful little games of making and breaking rules surrounding booze, such as only drinking on weekends, or only drinking every other day, or only drinking while doing a headstand naked.

What's trickiest about the grey area is that it's so socially accepted. It seems like everybody is in it somewhere, and the more normalized something becomes the less we think we need to change it. Safety in numbers, right? Every time I questioned my drinking I could point to at least ten people I know who drink way more than me, and as a chronic overthinker I was never sure if my concerns were legit or if I was simply overdramatizing everything as per usual.

When you listen and look around you, it's no wonder that it seems completely normal – even *necessary* – to drink. People have been drinking through the Trump administration, the pandemic, and to cope with discrimination, mansplainers, the patriarchy and childhood trauma.

In fact, one of my go-to comments was "I can't stand this without alcohol", and we all laughed and laughed. Fights with the husband, having to deal with annoying people, stress at work, a regularly occurring existential crisis, or even just an untidy house were all more than enough reasons to *wine about it*.

I've always been most interested in alcohol's medicinal qualities. I needed something to quiet the voices in my head for a while, to numb my overactive imagination and to relax. I don't perceive myself as a tightly wound person, but when I mentioned that to my husband he laughed out loud. "You are one of the most tightly wound people I know, babe," he told me, and while I argued the point, secretly I have to admit that he might be right. Sitting still and just *being* is not exactly my strength (he just burst out laughing again as I read him this sentence and unhelpfully added "that's an understatement"), and I always thought that having a few drinks helped me with that.

But now I'm learning that I couldn't have been more wrong. I'm fascinated by the connection between brain chemistry and alcohol and how interrelated the two are.

Experts say that a predilection towards drinking can come from an imbalance of neurotransmitters in the brain, which I have thanks to my mental illness. The cycle I've found myself in is the classic chicken-or-egg scenario:

I don't have enough serotonin in my brain, which is a natural antidepressant neurotransmitter.

Low serotonin=low mood.

For that reason I take an artificial antidepressant called an SSRI, a selective serotonin reuptake inhibitor.

The thing with the SSRI is that the effect is subtle. You don't get a high from it; it's more of a levelling out. You don't experience the devastating lows anymore, but you're also not experiencing the thrilling highs.

That's where booze comes in. Taking that first sip of delicious wine, a rush of euphoria would flood my body and transform that low mood into a better, more elevated one. Yay! That's thanks to a release of dopamine, the pleasure neurotransmitter. Dopamine lives in the brain's reward centre, and when we do something that gives us pleasure we boost our dopamine levels.

High dopamine=high mood.

Sounds awesome, right? Sadly, there's a downside: if we drink regularly, the body gets used to the alcohol and doesn't stimulate the dopamine as easily anymore. Translation? We need more booze to get the same dopamine rush, and we crave that dopamine rush because we are feeling depressed without it.

The culprit for this unpleasant side effect is called the hedonic set point[12], our "pleasure baseline". It's the place where our brain receives enough dopamine to feel a pleasure response. If we drink regularly and flood our system with high levels of dopamine all the time, this baseline rises over time. This means that we need higher levels of dopamine to feel pleasure, and here comes the worst part: things that naturally boost our dopamine levels – sleep, sex, lying in the sun, exercise, hobbies – can't reach the elevated threshold anymore. Eventually, the only thing that reaches our pleasure threshold and makes us feel good is alcohol.

But here comes the real kicker: our body craves a state of homeostasis. If your grade 12 biology is failing you, here is the simplest definition: staying in balance. When the body is out of homeostasis it enters a state of allostasis (= process that maintains homeostasis) to re-establish balance.

That means when we have a surge of dopamine, our body is out of

---

[12] Dopamine and the Hedonic set Point, Reframe app

balance and will immediately start working towards getting back into balance. How? By releasing GABA (gamma-aminobutyric acid), an inhibitory neurotransmitter which reduces energy, slows down your brain and calms you down. GABA is also the one to blame for your stumbling, slurring and increased clumsiness when you're drunk.

If you drink regularly, your body knows that a steady supply of alcohol will keep stimulating GABA receptors. As part of allostasis it adjusts by setting a new, lower set point of GABA to maintain homeostasis. This is fine as long as there is alcohol coming in to drive the last few GABA receptors hard. But if it stops, there is suddenly not enough inhibition in the system, which means not enough of a calming effect.

Low GABA=increased anxiety, agitation, anger, and dysphoria (feeling generally down and dissatisfied with life).

With a decrease in GABA we are in a constant state of tension. Our brain, knowing that alcohol will temporarily (!) relieve that tension by stimulating GABA will send cravings that tell us to have that glass of wine because it will make us feel better. Cruelly, while one glass may help GABA it won't do anything for the dopamine release we are accustomed to. We are long past the point where one glass does it. So we keep on drinking, chasing that lovely dopamine rush, because without it we are feeling depressed. This in turn decreases GABA which puts us into a state of anxiety.

To summarize: we drink when we are depressed to get the high from the release of dopamine. With too much dopamine in the body we need GABA to balance it out. Regular drinking reduces GABA, which leads to anxiety and generally feeling shitty. This depresses us and remembering that once upon a time drinking made us feel amazing we reach for the bottle, chasing that high ever more desperately by consuming ever more glasses. Which in turn leads to more anxiety ...

A vicious cycle if there's ever been one.

People with depression are at a higher risk for substance abuse and addiction and learning the brain chemistry behind it explains why. We use it as medicine, wanting to numb the voices in our head, craving the short-term dopamine rush without realizing the long-term negative effects on our mental and physical health. **It's much easier to see the correlation between drinking and feeling good in the moment than it is between drinking and feeling terrible in the long run.** There are so many other culprits who could be responsible for my increasing anxiety and worsening depression: the fucked-up state of the world, the misogyny, the pandemic, global warming, the ignorance and lunacy of people – it's not hard to find reasons to be depressed and anxious about.

Drinking makes everything so much harder instead of better though. It's not easy to see, not only because of the pleasant short-term effects but also because alcohol is being advertised so aggressively as the ultimate relaxant, de-stressing tool and essential party accessory.

That's the deviousness of alcohol: it seemingly provides the crutch to help us through the problems that have been caused by alcohol. It's like having a toxic friend who makes our life hell and then going to that toxic friend for help.

I read that quitting drinking is an excellent antidepressant and anti-anxiety treatment, and even after just a few weeks I can feel a difference in my mental health. I feel – lighter, somehow. Less weighed down. I feel a million different things all at once, and it's pretty exhausting to be honest. Once you turn off the steady supply of numbing agent, the world comes flooding back around you, and it's suddenly in technicolour and with the volume turned all the way up. I'd never noticed that I had put a nice protective wall of glass around me that kept me distanced from the world. I saw everything and the world saw me, but I was separated from it. My five senses were numbed by the glass, and the colours, smells, voices, sights, and smells were muted. Now the glass is gone, and I'm exposed to so much stimulation that I'm overwhelmed by it.

I feel like Sleeping Beauty who's just woken up after a nice, 100-yearlong nap.

Time to rediscover the world sober.

The Goopy Stage

I love butterflies. Spotting the first one in the spring always gives me a huge jolt of joy, and I smile every time I see them dancing in the sun.

Now I have another reason why I'm fascinated by them: I want to find out more about the process of becoming a butterfly. I have a vague idea that they turn from eggs into caterpillars into butterflies, and that the transition phase is called metamorphosis. But what exactly *happens* during the metamorphosis? My interest is more than just scientific – it's personal. I'm going through my own metamorphosis, and let me tell you, it sucks.

Caterpillars can relate. Once they've partied their socks off by eating their weight many times over it's time for prison. To add insult to injury, they have to make their own prison, the pupa, and seal themselves in it. It's like digging your own grave, isn't it? I guess the upside is that they get to decide where the couch goes and what colour the walls have, so that's something.

Once they've locked themselves into their pupa (also known as the chrysalis), the messy part starts. And as with so many unpleasant parts of life, this one is hidden away from the world. Luckily there are people like me who want to explore and share the raw and ugly and real parts of life, and they've provided us with details of what's going on in the chrysalis. Let's just say this upfront: it ain't pretty. The caterpillar's body digests itself from the inside out, using the same juices it used to digest food to now break down its own body. What a goopy mess!

No wonder they don't want to show that shitshow to the neighbours. But it's also oddly comforting because quitting alcohol is goopy as well.

I don't have to deal with physical withdrawal symptoms and I'm very grateful for that. I've seen a few patients come through the ER over the years in active withdrawal, and it's scary. Symptoms that are considered minor include tremors, anxiety, nausea and vomiting, and insomnia. Patients in that state are a twitchy, sweaty mess, in terrible physical and mental pain, and I'll never forget how a grown man sobbed his heart out to the doctor, telling him how he wanted to quit and just couldn't do it. And that's considered "minor" symptoms. The really bad shit is delirium tremens, better known as DTs, which present as severe confusion (think: you don't know your own name, where you are or what's going on), seizures, and autonomic hyperactivity (dangerously high blood pressure, fast and irregular heartbeat, intense sweating, abnormally high body temperature) – you're basically a human pressure cooker about to explode. DTs are very dangerous because they can end deadly. That's why it's vital for people with alcohol abuse disorder to withdraw under medical supervision – otherwise they might die.

I remember how shocked I was when a nurse told me that alcohol is the toughest drug addiction to overcome with the worst withdrawal symptoms. "Worse than heroin?" I asked in disbelief.

"Oh yes," she replied. "People don't die of heroin withdrawal even if it may feel like they do; but they can die of alcohol withdrawal." I was stunned. I'd had no idea.

While I don't have physical withdrawal symptoms I do experience cravings all the time in the beginning. There is a reason for that: neuroplasticity.

Neuroplasticity refers to the brain's miraculous ability to change and adapt to new information. The brain is always learning, and it creates new learning pathways based on that information. It creates paths in the brain, and the more we use the path the bigger and more easily to use it gets. My brain unfortunately learnt that alcohol equals a surge of dopamine, which equals pleasure. As a result it strengthened the path so much that it turned into a fucking highway, leaving the other, less travelled roads such as yoga or napping to grow over and slowly fill up with weeds.

Every time I needed some pleasure, my brain signaled me to "drink! It's the quickest way to the promised land!" And I happily obliged.

But now that I've entered uncharted waters my poor brain doesn't know what to do at first. It tries to lead me to the nice, big highway, the fastest way to some fun and relaxation, and I'm simply not following orders. What's a brain to do? **It starts to adapt and change again!** Neuroplasticity for the win. I'm no martyr for the cause, and with alcohol removed from my life I do my best to give my body and brain as much pleasure as I can in different form. I rediscover my love for chocolate (I lost it in the ocean of wine of the last few years), I read and read and read (that's always been my favourite drug), I write every day, I watch TV with my husband for hours, and I sleep more than I have in years. Oh God, the sleep! The sleep is a revelation. It is so magnificent; it almost makes up for the misery of missing wine.

I've read in every single quit-lit book how much better the sleep gets, and hallelujah, they were not lying. I sleep through the night and wake up refreshed every single morning. I take naps almost every day after I get home from work, falling asleep in under five minutes and waking up feeling great. Sleeping is like a drug to me, and I swear I can feel my entire body sighing with relief and gratitude that I finally give it the rest it has needed for so long.

Mornings are glorious now. My favourite time of day has always been the early morning – I naturally wake up between 5 and 6 am, but battling a hangover spoiled it for me. Now I have my mornings back: drinking coffee in bed with the dogs sprawled out all around me, writing or reading or meditating, and checking in faithfully with my sobriety app *Reframe*.

I downloaded it a week into my new life because I realized that I needed all the help I could get, and a tool to keep me accountable is essential. Aside from Richard and my sister nobody knows yet that I've quit, and they're both still drinking. I'm all alone doing this, and I need some emotional (and practical) support. Those nifty tidbits about the hedonic set point and neuroplasticity? I learnt them on *Reframe*. It gives you daily readings about the psychology behind alcohol, tools to help you battle through cravings, meditation prompts, a community of like-minded people and regular health updates. It also counts the days (and hours) since your last drink and tells you how much money you're saving. I spend less than ten minutes on it every day, but it really helps.

Because here is the uncomfortable truth: despite the beautiful mornings and superb sleep I miss wine. I've never been aware that I have triggers for drinking, but now I get to know them all in painful detail: coming home from work, cooking, days off, being bored, feeling down, feeling happy, feeling frustrated, feeling angry, making a fire, celebrating something, having friends over, talking to my sister on the phone, watching certain TV shows, hearing someone talk about wine. Even the fricking wine emoji is a trigger, and let me tell you, it's being used a *lot*.

It's an uncomfortable eye-opener just how much alcohol has infiltrated every aspect of my life. In that first month I grieve the loss of wine like the loss of a close friend. It is a toxic friend, yes – but how much fun we've had over the years! I reminisce about long, intimate talks with my husband around bonfires, fuelled by endless drinks; I get misty-eyed when I remember how we drank away an entire afternoon in a bar in Hawaii until we got cut off and asked to leave; I cry just thinking about how I will never drink with my sister again like we did in London, Paris, and in each other's houses. What am I doing? Why do I want to make my life so unnecessarily hard? Am I a masochist who *wants* to feel bad? My drinking is fine, isn't it?

Fortunately, I have written down a list of stuff that happened while drinking, and I pull it out every time alcohol tries to lure me back with its one-sided recollections of the great times we've had. That list is sobering (pun intended): the fights I had with Richard, passing out, falling down the stairs at a friend's place, burning my arm because I was drinking while cooking, falling off a horse, driving when I shouldn't, the 2am wakeups, the tearful phone calls with friends when a problem I had was a thousand times magnified by booze, the hangovers, the self-loathing, the fear. Oh God, the fear: I was terrified that I was doing irreparable damage to my liver, my stomach, my brain, and my mental health.

So I make myself the hundredth cup of peppermint tea, unwrap another bar of chocolate and cling onto the much-repeated refrain that "it will get better".

And it does with the arrival of month two. I'm feeling fantastic! I have tons of energy, my sleep is still excellent, and not drinking suddenly feels like a breeze. I've read about the pink cloud, a honeymoon period of early sobriety where you feel on top of the world, and I'm thrilled that I'm getting to experience it. It feels a bit like being in love, which I guess is true – I'm in love with my new life. My mental health is thriving, and I can't imagine ever feeling down again. My books warn me that this feeling won't last, just as no honeymoon period lasts forever. This high is not sustainable, but I'm enjoying the hell out of it while it's here. I'm living in the moment, baby!

I'm so pumped that I decide to do something terrifying: I'm telling my therapist Lola that I quit drinking because I used to drink too much. The relief I feel after unburdening myself of that heavy secret is indescribable. I gloss over the gnarly details (one step at a time), but even just saying it out loud to a relative stranger feels massive.

Brené Brown writes: *"Shame needs three things to grow exponentially in our lives: secrecy, silence, and judgment."*

I can confirm that this is correct. My drinking has been my biggest shame and my darkest secret, and the shame absolutely *thrived* in the environment of secrecy I created for it.

What makes shame so powerful is that it makes us believe that we are alone. And we are, because it cunningly prevents us from opening up to another person by convincing us that what we are hiding is so unspeakably terrible that people would despise us if they knew. So we stay silent, judging ourselves and truly believing that we are unlovable.

The way out of the shame cycle is having to do something that's incredibly difficult: opening up to someone. Brené Brown says that the antidote to shame is empathy. *"Shame cannot survive being spoken. It cannot survive empathy."* Easier said than done. You have to do the thing you are most scared of, which is risking someone else's judgment and possible contempt.

I was never brave enough to open up about my secret shame while I was drinking, but I am doing it now. The result is better than I could have imagined. I feel lighter, relieved, and – dare I say it? Proud of myself. That's not a sensation I'm very familiar with, but I like it. I like it a lot.

One day around the end of month two I come home from work and crave peppermint tea instead of wine. I can't believe it! It's a major win that makes me dance around the kitchen and whoop loudly – and evokes for one surreal, crazy moment the impulse that I should celebrate this win with champagne. It's a knee-jerk reaction that I have without thinking about it, because I've associated celebrating with champagne my entire life. Habits, man! Luckily I let that thought go right away, but not before recognizing the insidiousness of alcohol. Society has really done a number on us in terms of glorifying alcohol, and I've never questioned it until now. Not wanting to be manipulated by Big Booze is a new but compelling reason for quitting – I want to be truly free and not being told what to do any longer. Women have historically been told by the entire world how to behave, and I'm not following their rules anymore. Is quitting alcohol a feminist act? I believe it is.

Month three comes with bone-deep exhaustion. The pink cloud has drifted off, and grey clouds take its place. Not only is my energy gone, but I'm also starting to get all sorts of unpleasant physical sensations: headaches (I never get headaches), stomach aches, joint pain, that awful fog that precedes a depressive episode. I also get a weird ringing in my ear that comes and goes, which I've never had before. I'm so tired that I'm afraid I might drift off to sleep during my long commute to and from work, and no amount of coffee is helping. It's never ideal to fall asleep behind the wheel, but it's especially bad timing when you're navigating a treacherous mountain road that you're already terrified of.

Tears have started leaking out of my eyes with no apparent input from me. I'm powerless against it, and quite frankly, it gets awkward sometimes. When I talk with my co-workers about the state of affairs in healthcare (which is as bad as any of us have ever seen it) my eyes start gathering moisture. I have to excuse myself a couple of times because I don't know how to explain why I'm crying. I have no idea why I'm crying! My tear ducts seem to have taken on a life of their own, and I'm just along for the ride.

I quietly cry as I'm driving through the fire-ravaged forests. It's winter, and the white snow creates a stark contrast to the black tree stumps that are all that's left from last year's excessive wildfires. I try to remind myself that fires mean not only destruction but also renewal and rebirth, but I can't get the hang of it. I'm grieving for what's lost and can't see anything positive about it.

On days when I'm feeling low (and lately, all my days seem to be of that variety) I'm inexplicably drawn to the sadness and pain of the world. I can't focus on anything but terrible news, particularly stories concerning healthcare, and there's no shortage of that: local news articles are popping up with unsettling regularity, highlighting the severe staffing shortage, the long wait times, and the unprecedented number of healthcare workers leaving the profession. It's a strange feeling to be on a boat where so many of your fellow passengers are jumping ship. You can't help but start questioning if you should follow. Do they know something you don't? Are you a fool for staying? But what will happen to our communities, our patients, our *country* if the healthcare system collapses?

The fact is undeniable that I don't enjoy coming to work right now. I have to force myself out of bed in the morning after hitting the snooze-button two, three, sometimes four times. And I'm not the snooze-button type. I usually wake up on my own, without needing an alarm at all, but lately it's almost impossible for me to drag my sorry ass out of bed. You would think that I'd recognize a depressive episode by now, but somehow it never ceases to surprise me. That bitch manages to catch me unawares every time. What, you? What are *you* doing here again?

The reason behind it is that I hope after every depressive episode that it was the last one. Especially this time, after I felt so great last month. And I've quit drinking! I have to admit that I hoped that my depression would quietly disappear once I stop feeding it booze, never to be seen again. This obviously isn't so. This episode has brought a few old friends along: anger, irritability, major fatigue, weepiness, and a new one – cynicism. Let me tell you, she's nasty. She tells me that the whole world is fucked, that everybody is just out for themselves, and that no matter what I do I won't make a lick of difference. I may as well give up and wait to die.

You think you're important? Cynicism taunts. *You can be replaced in a heartbeat. You think that you've done something important over the last two years? That you are a healthcare hero? You're delusional. That's just propaganda from the Big Man to keep you dancing. They're pulling your strings and you're too goddamn stupid to notice. They don't give a shit about you. Time to wake up, sweetheart.*

Oof. I try not to listen, to ignore it, but my defenses are down. Cynicism is pushing all my buttons, knowing all my insecurities and fears, and she's playing with me like a cat with a mouse. What that does to me is that I'm turning around and wielding cynicism as a weapon myself. I seem to have misplaced all my compassion and empathy towards patients, who are suddenly nothing but a giant pain in my ass. I can just about keep it together in front of them, but I roll my eyes behind their backs, give the closing door they've just exited the middle finger and mutter obscenities under my breath when out of earshot. It's shocking what I'm doing, but I can't stop. I usually love my job and my patients – what's happening? Am I possessed? Do I need an exorcism?

"You're burnt out," Lola says matter-of-factly during the emergency session I've called. I just spent twenty minutes sobbing, trying to explain everything that's been going on.

"B-b-burnout?" I stammer. "But my job isn't that bad, I don't even really work fulltime, I'm doing enough selfcare ..." I peter out, not knowing what else to say.

"Burnout is not a failure," Lola tells me firmly. "You've been under too much stress for too long. Let me ask you this: you know other people who've burnt out, don't you?"

I do. We've talked about it before, because Lola treats quite a few healthcare workers and we've both mentioned how many of the people we work with had to take stress leave due to burnout.

"Do you think any less of any of them?"

"Of course not!" I exclaim. "I totally get it, everybody deserves a break!"

She looks at me meaningfully. "Including you, Miriam."

I'm silent for a moment.

"But how do you know it's burnout? Maybe it's just my depression?"

"Let me ask you a few questions. Are you tired all the time?"

I nod.

"Do you dread going to work?"

I nod again.

"Do you feel detached from your work?"

I consider this. "Do you mean that I don't enjoy work?"

"Yes, but more than that: do you become annoyed or irritable more easily than usual?"

I laugh for the first time that day. "You could say that. I'm actually scarily annoyed with everything right now. It's so bad that I was genuinely afraid the other day that I was gonna yell at a patient."

Lola grins. "Oh dear. What did he do?"

I make a dismissive hand gesture. "Oh, you know. 'COVID isn't real, the government is tracking us with the vaccine', all that bullshit. I shouldn't let it bother me, but I'm just so sick and tired of having to listen to every person's stupid opinion. I wish I could just tell them to 'shut up, please'."

"Well, there are ways: you could say that you don't want to discuss it. Tell them you don't talk about COVID. Or don't answer. Just because they're talking to you doesn't mean that you are obligated to reply."

"That never occurred to me!" I say in astonishment. "I always think that it's impolite to not keep a conversation going."

"Fuck that," Lola blurts out, and we both laugh.

"Women have been conditioned to be nice and polite, but that's the patriarchy talking. Men do it all the time. Have you never noticed women making polite small talk and men being too busy to answer, and nobody questions it?"

"All the time," I nod.

"Exactly." Lola switches gears. "Okay, back to burnout. I have one more question for you: do you feel like you're less productive at work lately? That you're using an enormous amount of energy and you still get little done?"

"Yes!" I pause to collect my thoughts. "Every little thing seems impossibly difficult. Making the decision to pick up the phone to call patients for appointments takes me hours sometimes. I just sit there, staring into space, trying to motivate myself to find the paperwork, pick up the receiver, and make that call. Some days I can't do it at all. It's like swimming through molasses all the time – everything takes a thousand times more effort than it should." I start crying again. "It feels like having a heavy blanket draped all over you. It makes it difficult to breathe, move, speak, and hear. I feel like I'm drowning. Or going crazy."

Lola looks at me kindly. "That's burnout. Your body is telling you that it can't continue like that. Listen to it. You need a break."

Two days later I've done everything that needs to be done to get time off work. My doctor and I have agreed on four weeks for now and to reassess in a couple of weeks. I've cried through the entire process, bursting into tears every time I have to talk to anyone about going on leave: my superiors, my doctor, my coworkers. I feel unhinged, but I can't stop it. I also experience massive guilt, and a profound sense of failure. I hope my mother won't find out; she would be disgusted by my weakness.

But then it's done. And suddenly I have four weeks ahead of me with no work. What now?

Keynote Speaker

The first week passes in a blur. I mostly stay in bed, and I sleep and sleep and sleep. Lily stays with me, her solid body providing warmth and comfort. When I'm not sleeping I take her for leisurely walks, trying to check in with myself like Lola taught me: how am I feeling? *What am I feeling?* I scan my body, and to my surprise I notice that my aches and pains have all but disappeared. I had noticed the stomach-ache dissolving as soon as I arranged the leave from work, but everything else slipped my consciousness. Now I'm becoming aware that my joints are pain-free, there's no ringing in my ears and the headache is gone as well. I'm actually feeling – *good*? At least physically. Mentally it's a different story. It feels like a storm is going off in my brain, wind howling and rain lashing, and I can't make out anything through the deluge. Am I sad, depressed, numb? I don't have a clue. All I can do is shelf the questions for now and get through the days moment by moment.

But I realize that I'm only functioning at 50%, max. I have to book a hotel room to stay at after a minor medical procedure Richard is getting, and I book it not only for the wrong day but also the wrong month. I don't notice until I get the confirmation email telling me that they're looking forward to seeing me in five weeks instead of tomorrow. What the hell? I've never done that before. I get it straightened out, grateful that I'm not at work right now, having to make decisions concerning patients.

Another day I'm in the shower shaving my legs (a major achievement in a depression). Once I'm done I turn off the water, climb out and start toweling off. As I'm getting to my legs I do a double take. What the ...? I've shaved one leg twice and the other one not at all! My left leg is smooth as a baby's bum while the right one sports a healthy ten-day stubble. I shake my head in bewilderment before taking care of it. Is that what it feels like getting dementia? It's very unsettling.

With the distraction of work and the numbing of alcohol gone I'm now confronted with myself, unfiltered. And I realize that I can't remember the last time I sat with myself without distractions. Our modern lives don't leave room for that. From the time we are kids we are given schedules: school, homework, sports, music lessons, after-school activities – even play dates are scheduled.

Little kids don't have to look out the window during car rides or entertain themselves anymore, they now have screens to look at. Waiting and not doing anything during that time used to be a daily occurrence: waiting in line at the grocery store, commuting on public transport or in one's own car, waiting for the water to boil or the coffee to brew, waiting at the doctor's office. People used to just sit and stare into space, lost in their own thoughts.

But now we can't stand sitting with our own thoughts anymore. As soon as we have an idle moment we whip out our phones, desperate for distraction.

The art of waiting patiently is in danger of becoming extinct, and it's a huge loss. If we can't stand being with ourselves, what does that do to us? It creates a disconnect that is difficult to endure. And since we've gotten used to avoid being uncomfortable, we will do anything to not have to feel our uncomfortable feelings: we numb, we distract, we consume.

Most of us who drink, or smoke weed, or eat, or online-shop compulsively do it as a nice little escape from reality – and ourselves. It's like taking a vacation from life and our own company without having to go anywhere, and we do it because life can be a lot. It's awful and amazing, boring and exciting, mundane and extraordinary. It hurts more than expected, and it's more unpredictable than we were told. It also holds possibilities that are bigger than we thought possible, which is exhilarating and terrifying. It's both better and worse than what we are prepared for.

Dimming the intensity of it feels good at first – until it doesn't. Until you're dimming life, light, and experiences so much that they're in danger of being extinguished completely.

Since I've decided to take the dimmer switch out of my life I'm feeling everything fully again: the highs, the lows, and the boring in-between, which may just be the most difficult to deal with.

But then something arrives in my email inbox that promises to make life a lot less boring.

"We are looking for people who are willing to share their experience with mental health at the 2022 CAMRT conference in Vancouver. If interested, please submit your story, and tell us why you want to be a part of our mental health panel".

It's an email from the Canadian Association of Medical Radiation Technologists (CAMRT), the national association for anyone who works in Medical Imaging. That includes x-ray, CT, MRI, Ultrasound, Nuclear Medicine, and Radiation Therapy technologists.

I stare at it, electrified. It feels like the invitation has my name written all over it.

The last time I read something that immediately called my name was the advert looking for ranch hands in Canada in 2002. Applying to it changed my life: I found my great love, my country, and after some trial and error my career and my passion.

Now, 20 years later, I'm feeling called again. If there's one thing I have extensive experience with it is living with mental health problems. I've talked about it quite a few times one-on-one, have written about it occasionally and have answered questions about what it feels like to have depression. People who have never had it can't imagine what it's like; if they're curious (or need to understand because they've lost someone due to mental illness) I do my best to explain it to them. But I've never spoken about it in front of an audience that's larger than two or three friends or co-workers. This would be completely different: this would be a real speech in front of hundreds of strangers. Can I do it? Do I *want* to do it?

The answer comes to me immediately and without hesitation: yes. Yes, I want to, and yes, I can do this. I've rarely been more certain of anything in my life. My mind made it up I write the following as my application:

When I first started out as an x-ray technologist, I spent a lot of time in the bathroom. I didn't have any digestive issues; I had mental health issues. But at the time I didn't know it. I thought my irrational anger/inexplicable bouts of tears/paralyzing fear was due to "normal" workplace stuff: normal annoying co-workers, normal feelings of being overwhelmed, normal sadness. I cried many tears and screamed many silent screams into my fists in those bathrooms, all while desperately trying to convince myself that this was "normal". I had been telling myself for close to 20 years that all those unsettling feelings of anger, rage, numbness, and despair were "normal".

Until my husband couldn't take it anymore. He was the one who convinced me to seek help. And I only did because he told me something that scared me to death: "I love you so much. But I don't know if I can stay with you if you don't try to get better." I didn't want to lose him. So we went to my GP, who was amazing. He listened, he understood, he made me feel seen. For the first time in my life, I didn't feel alone. That was in 2012. I've been on anti-depressants since, and I started therapy in 2020.

In addition to depression I've also been diagnosed with PMDD and anxiety. Talking about it in therapy and everyday life has helped me tremendously. I write and talk very openly about my mental health issues, and the most common response I get is this: "I feel the same." "Thank you for sharing." "It's great not to feel alone." "Thank you for opening up." I've been an x-ray technologist since 2010, and I love my job. But I've cried about patients. I've grieved for co-workers who suddenly passed away. I've felt demoralized by a public who seemed to have suddenly turned against us. I've experienced burnout and had to go on stress leave. I sometimes feel discouraged – or pissed-off – when the public doesn't acknowledge our existence by not even bothering to learn about our profession. But I've assembled an invaluable assortment of tools that help me navigate my mental health challenges. I'd love to share them with you.

I read it over once and then send it off before I can change my mind.

A few weeks later I receive the reply congratulating me for having been chosen as one of three panelists for the mental health panel.

I read the email once, then twice, and then I gently close my laptop and gaze out of the window. If I want to back out, now's the time. There were a lot of submissions, so it won't be a problem for them to find someone else if I decide not to participate. But if I accept then I'm really going all in: I will make mental illness part of my story, in front of my professional peers.

A deep calm settles over me as I realize how much I want to do this. I want to take part in the movement that will make it more acceptable to be someone with mental illness. I want to be the change that will make talking about mental health as normal as talking about the common cold. I'm also excited that my profession finally recognizes the importance of mental health, and I want to help spread the word. I know how desperately needed the larger conversation is.

I've lost friends to suicide caused by depression. I've seen too many people trying to drink or smoke or snort or eat their pain away. Hell, I'm one of them myself.

But if I stand there in front of hundreds of people and tell them that "hey, I'm a woman with anxiety, depression and PMDD", I have to embrace this part of myself and finally fully accept it. More importantly, I have to accept it as the active part it is, and not pretend it's a little problem I used to have.

I often tell the story of my mental illness as if it all happened in the past. I like to give the audience a happy, hopeful ending, the classic "it was bad then but it's great now and I live happily ever after". It's wishful thinking, but I secretly hope that if I tell it like that often enough it will come true. If I just get the knack for meditation and write often enough in my gratitude journal and do my breathing exercises and maybe put a few crystals on my nightstand then it will be over for you, bitches!

But the evidence suggests otherwise. While medication, therapy, mindfulness, and all the other big and small things I do help tame the dragon that is my mental illness, my dragon is still alive. And I'm beginning to think that it's never completely going to disappear.

Am I ready to tell them that?

The weekend of the convention dawns bright and sunny. The cherry blossoms are in full bloom, and with the sun sparkling off the water as I cross the Burrard Street Bridge Vancouver is looking pretty as a picture. I'm not speaking until tomorrow, but as I'm walking into the hotel I have butterflies in my stomach. In just 24 hours I'll have to stand in front of 550 people (the organizers are thrilled at the turnout) and tell people that I'm a bit mad in the head. Great.

I hesitantly approach the sign-in desk. It's still quiet since I'm very early, and three heads turn into my direction simultaneously.

"Hi," I begin tentatively.

"Are you Miriam?" one of the ladies behind the table asks me with a big smile.

"Yes I am," I say in surprise. Between the mask and my bangs only my eyes show. "How do you know?"

"I'm Val," she beams. "I'm one of the organizers and I recognize you from your photo. I'm so excited to meet you! We are all looking forward to the mental health panel tomorrow. It's one of our keynote sessions and interest is huge! Here is your badge," she hands me a large, laminated name tag that has a green ribbon with the word "speaker" attached to it. It looks very snazzy. I swallow and put it around my neck.

"And here's your swag bag," she continues and hands me a bag filled with goodies. "See ya later!"

Dismissed, I clutch the bag tightly to my chest as a shield and walk away, not knowing what to do next. I briefly consider checking out the vendors that have set up their booths, but tears are starting to fill my eyes. My heart is beating rapidly, and I'm suddenly feeling nauseous. *I have to get outta here*, I realize in a panic, and I look wildly around. I came up in an elevator, but there's no way I can go into a tightly enclosed space right now. I start speed-walking, hoping to find an exit asap before I start sobbing hysterically in the middle of the hotel. Luckily the hotel is all glass, and within seconds I spy escalators leading to an exit a floor below and almost run to them. I step out into a leafy courtyard with more cherry trees and benches dotted around. A group of tourists is walking past, chattering excitedly. It's very peaceful, but I'm shaking all over, so I sink down onto a bench and close my eyes.

Lola has taught me voo breathing, a breathing technique designed to calm the nervous system by stimulating the vagus nerve. It's simple: you take a deep breath in, and when you slowly breathe out you say "voo" in as deep a voice as possible, mimicking a foghorn The first time you do it is awkward, but boy does it ever work. I quietly voo for a minute. My heart rate slows down and my tears stop. I open my eyes and look up at the blue sky. I feel tiny and insignificant, and completely nuts for having volunteered to do this tomorrow. It seems insurmountable. What if I burst into tears and can't speak? "Don't think about it now," I tell myself. "That's future-Miriam's problem."

I get up and walk around for a bit, taking slow, calming breaths. Then I buy myself a coffee and head back inside. It's half an hour before the start of the conference and the noise level has increased considerably. There are a lot more people milling around now, drinking coffee, eating breakfast, talking, and laughing. I find a quiet spot by a window and sit down, continuing to take slow, deep breaths. A few feet away from me stands a woman who is digging through her purse. I glance at her briefly and then do a double take. "Kim? Is that you?" The woman looks up, and after a moment of incomprehension she recognizes me as well. "Miriam! How nice to finally meet you!"

Kim is the facilitator of our panel tomorrow. We've had a few Zoom meetings together with Taylor and Steph, the other two panelists, and I'm delighted to see her. "I'm so happy to see a familiar face! I almost had a panic attack just now about tomorrow. It's really happening, isn't it?!" I babble.

"I can't tell you how much I admire your courage to share your story. It's very brave. We really appreciate what you three are doing."

"Oh!" I'm taken aback by that. I didn't expect a thank-you, but it's nice. "I'm excited – and freaked out – to do this. But maybe wait until after the discussion before you thank me, I have no idea how it will go. I'm really nervous. But I know how important it is, and I'm happy to be here!" As I'm saying it I realize that it's true. The butterflies aren't a bad thing; they're a sign that I really care.

"Kim? Miriam?" A young woman in a black suit rushes to us and envelops me in a hug. "I'm Steph! I'm so excited to finally meet you in person!"

We greet each other enthusiastically, and a minute later we are joined by Taylor, the fourth woman to complete our panel. We've all made it, and even though I don't know these women we are united by a common goal: to help get one step closer towards ending the stigma of mental illness. This is really happening – and I'm not nervous anymore. I'm exactly where I'm supposed to be.

We attend the morning sessions, have lunch together, and then go over tomorrow's presentation. It's an hour long where we will share our story and then answer questions from Kim, mainly about mental health in the context of our profession. Feeling better and as well prepared as I'll ever be Taylor and I decide to skip the next presentation and have tea together.

We've hit it off right away. It's wonderful to talk to someone who gets it. This is the first time in my life that I've met someone with a similar mental health history, and it feels incredible to be able to exchange war stories without having to explain anything. We talk about the strain our mental illness puts on relationships, about what helps and what doesn't, about working in a care-giving job when you have a mental illness.

"It definitely helps to empathize with the patients," Taylor says, and I nod in agreement.

"It just takes everything out of us and leaves us in a puddle on the floor some days," I add, and we both laugh.

"I can't tell you how much box breathing I've done at work," Taylor says, referring to a breathing technique where you breathe in to a count of four, hold the air in your lungs for a count of four, exhale for four and keep your lungs empty for four. It's a well-known calming technique that helps to lower stress and decrease panic. Navy SEALs apparently do it, which makes it a lot more appealing. Who would have thought that we have something in common with Navy SEALs?

"My co-workers don't understand how I can struggle with my mental health and at the same time be willing to publicly speak about it in front of 550 people," she tells me, and I nod again. I get it. It seems contradictory to do public speaking, something many people are terrified of, while having anxiety. But here's the thing: Taylor and I are both pros at doing things that scare us. We do it all the time. We are used to forcing ourselves to show up at work on days when we think we can't do it, we go to parties we don't want to go to, we show up at therapy when we think we don't have it in us.

People with mental illness aren't weak; **we are the strongest motherfuckers you'll ever meet**.

The world is much scarier to us than to someone without a mental illness, but we still show up. We may be doing it with weak knees and a shaking voice, with a racing heart and tears streaming down our face, but we do it again and again and again.

Speaking up for our people at this conference is important to both of us. We want to set the record straight, to dispel some of the misconceptions, and to be a voice for the many of us who haven't found their voice yet.

There's another reason why we're doing it. Taylor is a confident, serene, successful woman who radiates warmth, kindness, and self-assurance. I would have never guessed that she struggles with the same demons I struggle with if I hadn't known.

I know that I come across as positive, cheerful, even bubbly. I *am* those things, just as Taylor is confident, warm, and self-assured. But we also have another side to us, a darkness that we hide from the world because that's what you're supposed to do: you don't worry or upset others, and the most important rule of all: you don't show weakness.

How many of the strong, capable, positive, and upbeat people you meet and work with and are friends with have days where they can barely make it out of bed? How many battle their own demons all alone, too afraid to confide in someone? **More than you know.**

They suffer in silence, making up socially acceptable excuses such as migraines or stomach aches or diarrhea for the days when they can't face the world, and when they can they return with their masks firmly in place.

The burden is heavy enough without having to hide it. The shame of mental illness flourishes only in the dark. We want to be trailblazers, to throw open the closed doors and let the light in, to show you that just because you have a mental illness doesn't mean that you can't also be successful, thriving, and happy.

These things are not mutually exclusive, no matter what they made you believe. We are multi-faceted, complex beings who can be many things at once – you are not one or the other, you are *all* of it.

That's what we tell the audience the next morning. Our eyes stay dry, and while our knees shake and our hands are wet with nerves, our voices are steady. I focus on a group of women in the front row who look kind and attentive, speaking mostly to them. They nod and listen, and at some point, their eyes are wet.

When we are done, the audience starts to clap. And then, one by one, they rise to their feet, giving us a standing ovation. It's surreal, and powerful, and beautiful.

Message delivered – and received.

Lily

The phone call comes on a Wednesday at work. I'm on my lunch break, just about ready to head back to the department, when Richard calls me. "Miriam, I have bad news. I'm so sorry ..."
I know before he even says the words. I burst into tears, my heart breaking. My baby is dead.

* * *

Christmas Eve, 2013
I come home from the late shift shortly before 1 am in the morning. Normally I'm tired yet wired, which I often treat with a glass of wine and a few episodes of *Friends* before going to bed. But tonight I'm wide awake, impatiently waiting for Richard and our youngest daughter Isabella to get home with a very special Christmas present.

At ten to two I finally hear the front door open.

"Do you have her?" I call as I fly down the stairs. Isabella cradles a small bundle in her arms, beaming. "Yes we do, look at her! She's sooo cute!"

A pair of bright, intelligent eyes looks at me curiously. She has a heart-shaped brown face, a black forehead, and two little white spots: one on her nose and one on her forehead. Most of her body is black, her front paws are white and her hind legs and undercarriage tawny brown. Her large bat-like ears stand straight up, giving the impression that she's wide awake and alert – an impression she'll live up to.

"Oh my goodness, come here puppy," I coo and take her from Isabella. The corgi puppy starts to immediately lick my face enthusiastically, and that's it: I'm hopelessly in love.

"What should we name her?" I ask the other two. She comes with the name Charlotte, but that's a lot for a little dog. We try a few names, until Isabella suggests Lily.

I look at the baby in my arms. "What do you think? Are you our Lily?" She looks up at me and starts licking my face again. "I think she likes it," I laugh, and it's settled.

I've always had dogs. My childhood dogs were Tina, a neurotic Dachshund, and Ronja, a hunting dog crossbreed with a fondness for taking off during walks and not returning until hours later. They were both typical family dogs, largely untrained and disobedient, and I loved them fiercely. The unconditional love dogs give you is a gift I've always treasured. If you have experienced conditional love, unconditional love becomes incredibly precious.

When I had my first major depressive episode at eighteen without knowing what it was, Ronja was the only friend who could make me smile. She was the only one who managed to pull me out: out of bed, out of my head, out of my despair. It would be another fifteen years before I received my diagnosis and my first prescription for antidepressants, but long before the pills I had the best natural antidepressants that exist: dogs. Medication and therapy and mindfulness are all necessary, but nothing has saved me as much as dogs have.

From the moment I moved to Canada we've always had at least three dogs at a time, often more. They were farm dogs, living and working outside, sleeping in kennels and the barn, looking after livestock. Richard grew up on a farm, and for a long time he was convinced that dogs were supposed to have a job. We had working dogs who loved being outside, and for many years that's how we kept our dogs. I would spend hours with the dogs outside every day, loving them and being loved in return.

Until Lily.

Lily has joined us for a special reason. At 34 years old I've just made the final decision on the Baby Question. Growing up I assumed that I would have a kid or two at some point in my life. Not so much because I have the burning desire, but because that's what you do as a woman. If you're married you have a baby, that's just how it is. I've never really questioned it, until the time comes that I have to make up my own mind. Aside from the fact that my husband is 25 years older than me and that I already have four stepdaughters, the big question I have to answer is this: do I *want* a child? Societal conventions and expectations aside, what do *I* want?

When I realize that I don't want children, it takes me a while to deal with the muddle of emotions that come up. Relief, sorrow, gratitude, mourning, peace of mind – I have to deal with them all. Even though I know that this is what I want, if you've thought that your life would go a certain way and then it doesn't, there is a normal grieving period you go through.

Am I relieved that I won't raise my own children? Yes I am. I've been a stepmom for eleven years at this point, I know how hard it is. But I also know how fun and rewarding it can be, so I'm working through my sorrow that I'll never experience this with my own baby. Still, the most prevalent emotion I feel is overwhelming relief. I'm so happy that I'll never have to go through pregnancy and giving birth, the endless sleepless nights, constant worry, never having a moment to myself, the expense, and all the kid-related stuff I find so tedious: team sports, children's birthday parties, the judgmental professional moms, school lunches, school runs, the competitiveness between mothers.

I'm in the midst of working through all these feelings when Richard meets a corgi at the feed store. It's the first corgi he's ever seen, and he's charmed by her intelligence, friendliness, and cute appearance. Despite the short legs, corgis have the body, temperament, and bark of a big dog. Their compact bodies are much more agile than you would think, and their little legs are powerful and muscular. With their large upright ears and bright eyes they miss nothing, and they're keenly alert watchdogs. Richard, who wants to help and save me as he has done countless times before, decides then and there to buy me a corgi.

As soon as he's home he gets on the Internet, looking for puppies. That turns out to be trickier than anticipated, with no corgi puppies available anywhere close to us. He eventually finds some in Pennsylvania in an Amish community. The owners Eli and Rachel use a broker for advertising and selling, and when Richard wants to talk to Eli, he has to call the only shared phone in the village at a certain date and time. The broker has sent a video of the puppies, and we choose Lily because she's the most adventurous and has a beautiful tri-coloured coat.

Since Pennsylvania is over four thousand kilometers away we arrange to get her flown to Vancouver.

And now she's here in the early hours of Christmas of 2013, eight pounds of ears and sass and confidence. The best part? She will be our first house dog. Corgis are herding dogs bred to move cattle, but Lily's job is to be my child and companion.

She will exceed all my expectations.

I bought a crate for her to sleep in and furnished it with a soft dog bed, blankets, and toys. We are expecting her to cry during the first night, missing her litter mates and her mother, but Lily inspects her new domain, curls up and promptly falls asleep. We kneel in front of her crate and watch her sleep. "I love her," I whisper to Richard. "She's the best Christmas present I've ever received."

"Good," he whispers back and kisses the top of my head.

Dogs choose their person. No matter what you do or how you bribe them, once they've decided who their number one is, that's it. They will love all the members of their pack, but none as much as the one they chose.

Lily chooses me. From day one she follows me around like a little shadow, keeping her watchful gaze on me at all times. I need to watch her constantly as well, because as it turns out, it's almost impossible to distinguish between her sitting down and squatting down to pee. Her fluffy butt hovers only inches above the floor, and even the smallest squat plants her bum right down. I never needed to potty train a dog before, but now I need to learn in a hurry. Little pee stains dot the carpet for a while, and the house starts to smell strongly of disinfectant. As soon as I see her getting ready to sit I cry "pee outside!" and lead her to the patio door. Poor girl doesn't get to sit down in peace for a while, but luckily she's smart and learns quickly. Instead of scratching on the door she talks to me. She will sit down in front of me, whine once, and then get up and turn around. If I don't follow right away she looks over her shoulder as if to say "what are you waiting for? Come on, I won't hold it all day!"

She's been sleeping in the crate and loving it, but one night the kids bring her into their bed. "She didn't move all night!" Isabella tells me excitedly the next morning, and obviously I have to see for myself. That night I don't lock her in, and she follows me into the bedroom and hops into bed as if it's the most natural thing in the world. She stretches out contentedly next to me, and after a while she turns on her back with her four little paws sticking straight into the air. Just as advertised she's a quiet and considerate sleeper, but the best part is that she stays in bed for as long as I'm there. It doesn't matter if it's 6am or 10, she doesn't move until I'm ready to get up.

We quickly become inseparable. I walk her daily, because corgis are energetic and athletic dogs that love to run and play. In fact, when I've been sitting on my computer for a while she will start asking to go out, gently at first but increasingly more insistent. She won't leave me alone until I give in, grab her leash and head to the front door. Overjoyed, Lily will run figure eights around and in between my legs as I try to put my shoes on, barking enthusiastically and nipping my legs to tell me to hurry up.

Her excitement is infectious, and once we are on our way I'm always happy she dragged me outside. But man, she can be infuriating. Independent and fearless, Lily does what she wants. When I call her it's more of a suggestion than a command in her opinion, and she often cocks her head and looks at me questioningly as if thinking it over before turning and trotting away from me when she doesn't feel like coming. Sometimes, that gets her into trouble.

One sunny afternoon in February we walk along the frozen river next to a little wooded area. Lily is off leash, happily hopping through the snow like a bottom-heavy bunny, having the time of her life. Suddenly she stands at attention, focused on something in the woods. A moment later she is off like a shot, scrambling through the deep snow of the ditch before disappearing between the trees. At first I'm not worried – a squirrel in a tree can inspire such a reaction. But when she doesn't come back after I've repeatedly called her name I sigh and start making my way towards the spot where she disappeared. I peer into the dark woods, and wouldn't you know it: she is right there, sitting about twenty feet away under a tree. "Lily, come here!" I call, but she just sits there, looking at me. I call again with the same result. Even for her that's weird. I get a bad feeling and start climbing into the ditch. It is a lot deeper than I anticipated, and I sink thigh-deep into the snow.

Using my arms to propel myself forward I wade as quickly as I can through the sticky snow, desperate now to get to my dog. Something isn't right. As I get closer I see something dangling next to Lily's head. What the hell is it?

And then realization hits me with a sickening jolt: it's bait. A deer foot is dangling from a string, and I'm terrified of what state I will find Lily in. Is she injured? Has she lost a leg, or worse?

She's still simply sitting there, motionless. She doesn't make a sound. "Mama is here baby, mama is here," I murmur when I finally reach her and I fall onto my knees, giving her a quick hug before carefully inspecting her body.

A thin piece of wire is trailing away from her, and I follow it to her body with trembling fingers. It's a snare trap, and the wire loop has caught her left hind leg. I gently pull off the sling and examine her leg, and to my enormous relief I see that Lily is uninjured. She seems just as relieved as I am about being freed and leaps up joyfully, licking my face in gratitude. Together we make our escape as quickly as possible. The west is still wild in some parts.

But having an adventurous dog definitely has its upsides. I take her everywhere with me: on car rides, ATV rides, in our canoe and my kayak. She comes snowshoeing and cross-country skiing, lies on my mat when I do yoga and hangs out in the hammock with me. When she can't come along she waits by the gate, ears pricked up alertly, keeping a watchful eye out for my car. As soon as she sees it her short tail goes into overdrive, and when I jump out of the car to greet her she dances in and around my legs in her signature figure eight, her lips pulled back in a (somewhat scary) corgi smile.

She's happy to do whatever I'm doing as long as she's with me. I've never had a dog who was so attached to me, and I say thanks for her every day.

Lily saves me on the bad days. When I can't get out of bed she snuggles close and won't leave my side. She doesn't ask for food or for a walk, wouldn't even go outside to pee if I wouldn't insist on taking her out, and no matter how long I stay in bed, she stays there with me. With her around I don't feel as lonely. Her love shows me that I'm worth loving, no matter how much the voices try to convince me that I'm unlovable. She doesn't do anything but being there with me, and that's all I need when I'm in a depression. That's all any of us need, depression or not: to have someone unwaveringly on our side, regardless how awful we think we are.

Dogs are the masters of unconditional love; no human being will ever come close.

She has an uncanny knack of knowing when it's time for me to get up and outside into the fresh air. Her ears will perk up, she will look at me bright-eyed and jump down from the bed, trying to motivate me to follow her. She's never wrong; when I eventually drag myself out the door and get going I always feel better.

I start bringing her to work with me, walking her before my shift and on my lunch break. I often take her inside so she can say hi to my co-workers, who all adore her. Lily loves people, and people love her. Being with a corgi in public is a bit like hanging out with a celebrity. People will point, smile, take pictures, and come up to us, wanting to pet her. She adores the attention, convinced it's nothing short of what she deserves. She's not wrong.

On a regular Tuesday morning I let her out to pee. It's a workday and I've planned to bring her along, but when I call her half an hour later she doesn't come. Lily likes to roam around the ranch, and when she's found something interesting – a chicken egg to eat, or a bone, or a particularly tasty piece of horse or cow manure – she ignores me. I shrug and drive off without her.

When I return in the late afternoon I'm surprised that she doesn't wait for me by the gate. As soon as I enter the house I ask Richard: "Where's Lily?"

"She had an accident today. I found her just outside the cow pasture; I think one of the cows stepped on her."

I'm alarmed. "Where is she? Is she okay?"

"She will be fine. I don't think anything's broken." He points me to her sister's crate in the spare bedroom. I race in and kneel down in front of her.

LILY

Lily looks as she always does, with no visible injuries. But she seems stunned, as if she can't quite believe what happened. She also doesn't get up to greet me, which is very unlike her. I carefully lift her out of the crate and carry her into our bed. She doesn't make a peep of discomfort, which reassures me. I stay with her for the rest of the day just as she does when I'm in bed. She doesn't have a fever and she doesn't seem to be in any pain. She doesn't move much, but I put it down to the shock of what happened and her maybe having a soft tissue injury on her leg. I resolve to bring her to the vet tomorrow if she isn't better.

The next morning I carry her outside to pee. She still doesn't walk, and now I'm freaked out. I have to go to work, so I tell Richard to bring her to the vet as soon as they're open. He does, and when he calls after the initial assessment I'm relieved: the vet agrees with us and doesn't think anything is broken. "She says that it's probably a soft tissue injury, and in a week or two she should be back up and running," Richard tells me. "They will do an x-ray just to be sure."

It will be a while before they do the x-ray, so they send Richard home, promising to call when Lily is ready for pickup.

My heart is a lot lighter as I go about my day, and I'm eager for Richard's call that will confirm that everything is okay. When his name appears on my phone screen towards the end of my lunch break I pick up after the first ring, expecting good news. What I'm not expecting is a long silence, and then his devastating words: "Miriam, I have bad news. I'm so sorry ..."

My heart plummets. I can feel it drop in my chest, and an icy chill crawls up my body. No. No no no no no – this can't be happening. I feel nauseous and tears start falling thick and fast before I can even utter a word. "W-what happened?" I stammer. "W-what's going on with Lily?"

Silence. I can tell through my panic and pain that he's trying to find the right words. "Babe, she's badly injured. Way worse than we thought – the vet was shocked. The x-rays show that her entire pelvis and part of her spine are smashed to pieces. She's paralyzed ..."

"But we can do surgery, right?" I interrupt. "They can fix it, can't they?"

"They can't do the surgery here, it's way too complicated. They don't think she has a chance anywhere else either. Even if she survives the surgery she would be incontinent for the rest of her life, paralyzed – it's no life for a dog."

I cry so hard now I can barely hear what he's saying.

"Are you sure? Are they sure? Is there really nothing we can do?"

"You have to let her go, honey," he says gently, and I cry harder.

"C-can you wait until I get there before they" – I can't bring myself to say the words *put her down*.

That's when another blow hits me. "It's already done," Richard whispers. "She was still sedated from the x-rays, and I told them to go ahead. She didn't feel a thing ..."

I howl like a wounded animal. The pain is as real as if I've been stabbed in the chest.

"I needed to be there!" I scream into the phone. "She needed me there! How could you? How could you not wait for me?"

"I'm sorry babe," he says quietly. "I did what I thought was best."

"I'm gonna go and pick her up. I want to bury her at home. Is she still there?"

He says she is, and I hang up. I tell my co-workers that Lily is dead and that I have to go, and then I walk straight out of work. Nothing in the world could keep me there a minute longer. Even though it's too late and my baby is gone, I have to be with her as quickly as possible.

I drive the hundred kilometers in a trance. I don't remember a thing about the drive once I arrive. I make my way into the waiting room like a sleepwalker, tears dripping down my chin. I tell the receptionist that I'm here to pick up Lily and that I want to see the x-rays, and she explains to me that the doctors are in a meeting and that I'll have to wait for them to be done. I go back outside to sit in my car and cry in private while I wait for the vet to come and get me.

When he finally does he's full of sympathy. He's not the one who treated Lily, but he's the one we know and like best. He shows me the devastating x-rays and I see that they've made the right decision.

"Can I take her home now?" I ask quietly, and he leads me into a back room. I'm expecting her to be in a box or something, but instead he goes straight to a large freezer.

"I'm sorry, I know this is macabre," he apologizes before opening the lid, "but unfortunately we get a lot of dead animals in a day." Then he opens up the freezer and reveals what's inside: black garbage bag after black garbage bag, filled with pets. For some reason that makes me laugh through my tears.

"Wow," I breathe. "I mean I get it, but it's still so unexpected." I can see that he regrets having brought me back here, but in a weird way I feel a bit better. It puts my loss into perspective. I'm not the only person who's lost a friend – this freezer full of dead animals proves that.

But when he picks a bag and I see the label "Lily Verheyden" on it I start crying again. He carries her out to my car, expresses his condolences one more time and then hurries back inside.

At home I take her out of the bag and gently lay her down in the rose garden next to my She Shed. Lily looks like she's sleeping. I sit down beside her, and while I stroke her soft fur I tell her how much she's meant to me. I tell her that she's been the best friend I could have ever wished for. I tell her that I love her, and that I'm so grateful for the past eight and a half years we spent together. I tell her that she's my baby, that I'll never forget her, and that she'll always be with me in my heart.

Then I get a shovel and bury my best friend in the world.

*　*　*

The moment you decide to get a dog you also invite future heartbreak into your life. With their average life expectancy of ten to twelve years in contrast to our 80 you will lose many dogs if you start early and never stop. I will never stop.

Love and grief come as a combo. You can't have one without the other. You could try to avoid grief by choosing a life without love, but that's way more tragic than loving and losing.

Richard and I usually have four dogs or more at a time, so we've lost a few in our twenty years together. It's painful every time, but to me, the heartbreak is the price you pay for all the love, fun and joy you get while you have your dog. It's a steep price, but it's worth it.

I grieve for Lily like no other dog before her. While I've loved them all, she was the most special.

And something else is different this time: I'm grieving without drowning my sorrows in wine. This is the first time since the loss of my childhood dog Tina that I don't use alcohol to help me through it, and to my great surprise it makes the sorrow easier to bear.

After previous losses I would cry into my glass night after night, becoming more distraught and beside myself with every drink. Instead of working through my grief I was numbing it, which set me back. It was almost as if I had to start the process of moving through my grief over again in the morning.

This time I'm fully present for all of it. While that sounds harder, it actually isn't. Because instead of getting tunnel vision that focuses solely on the loss, I'm also reliving the many happy memories I have, and while I cry every day I also smile and feel overwhelming gratitude for the time she and I had together.

Lily taught me to be joyful and to live in the moment. I will honour her by doing just that.

Surviving and Thriving with Mental Illness

From the moment I received the diagnosis of depression on a rainy November day in 2012 I was looking for a solution. At first I thought I got it right then and there: the simplified explanation of my kind doctor that a pill could regulate the hormone imbalance in my brain sounded to me like it would fix this annoying little problem I had.

This didn't happen. The strategy I used for the first few years – take a pill and pretend the depression doesn't exist – didn't work, annoyingly enough.

But I didn't want to deal with it beyond popping a pill every morning. I didn't want to go to therapy (what for? Everything was *fine*), and I certainly didn't want to change a single thing about my lifestyle. Did I know that alcohol was known for worsening depression and increasing anxiety? Sort of – didn't everybody? But I took it about as seriously as the warning on the little leaflets in tampon boxes that tampons could cause toxic shock syndrome. Do you know anyone that happened to? Yeah, me neither.

When I talked about my depression I always made it sound like it was a problem I used to have in the past that had been resolved. Depression cured! I couldn't accept it as a condition that kept affecting my life and the life of the people around me, and that had to be dealt with properly. Why? Because I didn't want to be someone with depression. I believed what society had taught me about mental illness: that it was synonymous with weakness, being crazy, being a liability. People with mental illness were not to be trusted. They couldn't be functioning members of society – they were a burden.

That could never be me. I wanted to be someone who was strong and resilient and brave. I didn't realize that having a mental illness and getting up every day, doing your best despite the war being fought inside your mind is nothing but bravery. It takes real strength and courage to face your demons over and over again.

But I didn't know that then. I spent a lot of time and energy needing to prove to everyone – and myself – that I was no different from "normal" people; that I was, in fact, one of them. Nothing to see here folks, just another regular hardworking and high functioning adult.

There's a reason why I avoided an official diagnosis like the plague and didn't seek help until I was on the verge of losing everything I loved. I knew something wasn't right with me long before that vacation in Hawaii in 2012, but I fervently hoped I could power through. Pretend it doesn't exist and maybe nobody else will notice it?

Taylor Tomlinson, a brilliant comedian whose Netflix special *Look at You* should be required viewing for everyone who has ever struggled with their mental health, talks about telling her friends about her diagnosis of bipolar disorder, and what one of them said to her upon finding out:

"Yeah, your mental illness was kinda like your middle name. I didn't know what it was, but I knew that you had one."

So much for thinking we can fool the people around us into not noticing our mental illness.

My entire life I've been trying to figure out who I am as a person. I've always been laughably clueless and unobservant about myself, not being aware of some pretty basic stuff: I never knew that I was an introvert until age 34, had never noticed that I have one floppy ear until Richard pointed it out, and it took me decades to finally learn that I get sick when I do too much and say yes too often.

But by far the biggest one is that I didn't want to acknowledge that mental illness is a part of me. It's a big, important part that can't be ignored. It's part of what makes me who I am. It will never go away completely. Acting like it doesn't exist, or like it's nothing more than a small nuisance does not serve me.

I refused to accept that. "I have mental illness, it doesn't have me," I'd blithely tell anyone who'd listen, feeling very clever. I tried to make everybody

– most of all myself – believe that having a mental illness was of no greater importance than the fact that I don't like cheese. Mildly interesting and baffling to some, but of no great importance.

After eight years of pretending – and failing – that my mental illness was nothing but a minor inconvenience I finally had to admit that faking it wasn't making it.

By acting like my mental illness was no biggie, I had done myself and the people around me a great disservice. It's like being lactose intolerant but still eating cheese all the time because it tastes so good, and everybody is eating it. Not only do you make yourself miserable, but the people around you also suffer. (I'm told the farting is grotesque. As is living with someone who has a mental illness but is in denial about it.)

Time for a new perspective. Funnily enough, it came from something my sweet doctor said back in 2012. He compared depression with diabetes in terms of it not being my fault. All I had to do was go one step further from there: if people with diabetes could learn to live with it, why shouldn't I be able to learn to live with mental illness? So far I'd been living against it; time to try a different approach.

The first thing I did was stop getting angry every time my husband asked me if I was about to get my period when I was acting irrationally. Just like Taylor Tomlinson's friend knew that she had a mental illness even if he didn't know the name of it, so did Richard know that my period was connected to my rage, intense mood swings and worsening depression I'm experiencing every month. That was long before either one of us had ever heard of PMDD, let alone knew that this is what I have. But every time he dared to utter the words "are you getting your period?" I would get absurdly mad. I was convinced that my rage was completely justified, that he was, in fact, *the worst and most annoying person alive*. How dare he suggest that it wasn't him but *me*? Ridiculous. I clung to my conviction with desperate stubbornness because what if he was right? What if it *was* me, and I was as awful a person as I had been led to believe? I didn't know that there was a third option: that it was neither him nor me, but a disease.

Even now I have to be careful to not to succumb to the knee jerk reaction of blaming Richard for everything, especially when my PMDD is alive and kicking. I've marked the danger zone (one week before my period) in my calendar in red ink and I check my period app every morning, so I know when the Mood arrives. Being prepared that my emotions aren't my own when my hormones go wild helps tremendously. I find that the best way for me to deal with my PMDD is to retreat from people as much as possible during the worst two days and to wait it out. That means that I'm quieter at work than usual, go outside into nature during breaks, and that I seek as much solitude and distraction as I can. I'll hide in stories in any possible form: by reading, listening to audiobooks, and by watching movies and TV shows. I also commiserate with friends who suffer from PMDD as well, which is cathartic. There is incredible relief and empowerment in the knowledge that you are not alone in something that can make you feel immensely ashamed and powerless. The more I share about PMDD, the more women approach me and say "I think I have it too! I thought I was just a bitch/going insane/not as tough as everybody else".

If we keep quiet about our struggles and health problems we're not only hurting ourselves; we also deprive other people from knowledge, a community, and the – possibly lifesaving – realization that they are not alone.

In chapter 9 I had to break the unfortunate news to you that there is currently no cure for PMDD except for menopause. To continue this series of unfortunate news, the same is true for depression. If you make the mistake I've made to google "is there a cure for depression?" you're in for a major disappointment. The consensus on the Internet is that the answer is no – there is no cure.

I refused to believe that. If I was still plagued by depression the only reason was that I hadn't found the right treatment yet. So I started trying different stuff: yoga in addition to my antidepressants, juicing, starting to go for regular walks with my dogs. I quit juicing after a few months (doesn't everyone?) and added more fermented grape juice instead.

I also tried to sit cross-legged on the floor, eyes closed, and meditate in total silence. This kind of meditation does not work for me but meditating during gentle movement does.

When I reluctantly added therapy (I do Cognitive Behavioural Therapy, CBT for short) I thought I'd cracked the code for getting rid of anxiety, depression and PMDD. Remember Tori's *Sedona Method* from chapter 14? It sounded like all I had to do was change my thinking from unhelpful to helpful, and Ta-da! I would be cured. Turn this frown upside down, therapy-style.

The Sedona Method didn't properly work for me because it over-simplifies the very complicated thought processes that occur in the brain of someone with anxiety and depression. However, its principle that psychological problems are based (in part) on unhelpful thinking is the same that CBT is based on, and I find that remarkably helpful.

Both Tori and Lola taught me that beliefs are thoughts we keep practicing. If we keep practicing ways of negative thinking they will lead to behaviour that's negatively impacting our lives, which then can turn into anxiety, depression, addiction, or destructive behaviour. CBT teaches you better ways of thinking, which translates into re-evaluating behaviour patterns, learning better problem-solving skills, developing greater confidence in oneself, and learning how to face and overcome fears. That's a long, hard road of two steps forward and one back, with some successes but also lots and lots of setbacks. I get the concepts in theory but applying them in real life is a different story. It requires self-awareness and patience, and patience has never been my strong suit.

"I thought once you've learnt all these skills you're set," I grumble to Lola during one session. "I really hoped that if you've solved a problem once you would never have to do it again. But instead I keep making the same mistakes, having the same fears, and needing to relearn the same lessons. It's like cleaning the same road over and over because it keeps getting dirty. It's so frustrating."

Lola points out that I am, in fact, making excellent progress, but that life has a way of throwing new problems our way.

This reminds me of the game Chutes and Ladders, an immensely frustrating game in my opinion. Even as a child I hated the randomness of it, the crushing disappointment when you were almost at the top, only to get kicked down to the bottom.

That game doesn't teach any skills (unless you count learning to be disappointed, in which case *well done*), it doesn't reward hard work or cleverness, and it certainly doesn't leave you feeling happy and relaxed.

The only lesson you learn is that life is random and unfair, and who needs to have that rubbed under their nose during play time?

For people with anxiety, the unpredictability of life is difficult to tolerate. That's why so many of us re-watch our favourite shows again and again, because we already know exactly what's going to happen and we don't have to fret and worry for a while.

To counteract the many things I can't control I've developed some strategies to help me get through life that make living with me challenging:

I need excessive reassurance: I ask my husband regularly if he still loves me and would like to ask my friends as well but feel too embarrassed to do so.

I use lists to help plan my day, at work, when making decisions, for my personal goals, for vacations, to remember the books I've read ... there are a LOT of lists in my life.

I find it difficult to delegate, especially to my husband, because I assume that he won't do it right.

I avoid situations that make me uncomfortable, especially social situations.

I frequently use distractions to mute the voices in my head.

Therapy has been helping a lot with my anxiety and depression, but I have come to realize that it won't cure me. And I have accepted that.

It has taken me ten long years to get to this point: ten years of denial, anger, bargaining, depression, and now, finally: acceptance. If these five words sound familiar it's because they are the often-repeated stages of grief. And I *was* grieving, even if a lot of it happened on a subconscious level. I was sad that I wasn't normal, mad that I had to deal with a mental illness as if life wasn't hard enough, I tried using relentless positivity against my mental illness, got discouraged when it didn't always work, and at last I have arrived here: accepting that this is my lot in life.

On the whole it could be a lot worse. I remind myself of that often when I make my gratitude lists and count my many blessings. I live a happy life filled with love, joy, fun, stories, friendship, laughter, and countless big and small moments of bliss. But I also have darkness, pain, and difficulty in my life, just as everybody does.

I'm always tweaking and adjusting what helps me live my best life, but if you want a list (and you're getting one, whether you like it or not), here are the most important tools in my bag of tricks on how to survive and thrive with mental illness:

- Antidepressants
- Therapy
- Daily walks (dogs optional, but highly recommended)
- Dogs
- No alcohol
- Plenty of sleep
- Daily dose of nature
- Books
- TV shows and movies
- Writing
- Lots of water
- Moving my body
- Kayaking (I meditate best in my kayak)
- Avoiding toxic people
- Taking mental health days when needed
- Listening to my body and mind
- Supplements
- Naps
- Hugs
- Hiding in bed when necessary
- Regular social interaction with people that fill you up (as opposed to drain you)
- Yoga
- Swimming in lakes
- Chocolate and candy

- Fresh fruit
- Bonfires
- Starry skies

This list isn't complete, and it's not set in stone. Some of its items have been on it since the beginning; others I've added more recently; some items have been removed because they weren't working (alcohol, I'm looking at you).

Life isn't set in stone. It's always moving, changing, fluctuating. It's not an easy concept to embrace for someone like me who overthinks everything, worries excessively and fears the future often. But the list helps. Having accepted that mental illness is a part of me helps. Hugging my dogs and my husband helps. Practicing mindfulness, aka living in the moment helps. And some days hiding in bed and re-watching *Call the Midwife* helps.

Sometimes I forget that pain, fear, sadness, and boredom are part of every life. We live in this strange world where we can choose which reality we want to live in: a curated, aggressively positive reality? Or one where we focus on everything that's terrible, unjust, and doomed? Do we choose not to believe anything we don't like to hear by declaring it "fake news"?

Or do we select a few people or sources and believe everything they tell us?

Do we want to trust in the basic goodness of people, or have we arrived at a place where we don't trust anyone?

For a while I was living in this strange in-between world where I was swinging wildly between thinking I was an eternal optimist and falling hard and fast into a deep pit of despair. Alcohol was a great helper in achieving that horrible roller coaster, but I'm pleased to report that I've stepped off this ride since I quit.

I'm still figuring stuff out: my mental health, the world we live in, people, life. I will never be done figuring it out because life is constantly changing. My goal is to change, grow and evolve alongside with it.

Because no matter how broken my brain and the world around it are at times, I'm sure of one thing: life is completely, breathtakingly beautiful.

Epilogue

I started writing this book six weeks after I quit drinking. The words came easily, eager to come out, and I finished the first draft after only five months, the fastest I've ever written anything. It was my way of processing the previous two years, which were immensely stressful, and to document in real time what it felt like to rediscover the world sober.

I'm afraid often. When you have anxiety, the world seems a scary, intimidating place, and being scared is part of my personality.

But 2021 was especially terrifying. While many of my regular fears are self-made (I know at some level that they exist only in my head), in 2021 the outside world turned into a place of constant danger and unpredictability. My co-workers and I were still traumatized from facing a virus we knew nothing about except for its ability to kill healthy people at random.

And suddenly there were dead children, fires that turned the sky dark and the world into an apocalypse, roads that were icy, on fire, swept away or closed before I could make it home. There was a flood that happened without warning and shut down our entire town for two weeks. On top of that, we were harassed at home (I chose not to write about it in this book) and my entire profession was harassed at work for trying to help people.

Nothing felt safe; danger was everywhere.

And there was this dark, heavy secret I was carrying around: my drinking.

I don't consider myself an alcoholic. Drinking wasn't an addiction for me – it was a habit (pushed heavily by society) that turned into a coping mechanism.

I desperately wanted to escape a reality I could barely cope with, and wherever I turned, alcohol was there: praised as the ultimate escape, treat, and tool to relax. Constant repetition of these messages sunk in so deep that it became automatic: my first impulse at signs of stress was that I wanted a drink.

I don't blame myself or anyone else for falling for it. Alcohol is considered a rite of passage, a normal – and necessary! – part of adulthood in our society. It's being heavily advertised constantly, and if you don't participate *you* will be seen as the one having a problem, when in truth our society is the problem for pushing an addictive substance and lying about its terrible health effects.

I didn't quit because I hit rock bottom. I quit because I deserved better. I wanted more: more peace, more time in my days, more creativity, more sleep, more adventure.

You know what? I found it all. Where 2021 was the year of fear, 2022 has been the year of strength. Quitting alcohol has given me countless gifts: I've accepted my mental illness, taken down bullies, become more empowered, talked in front of 550 people, found our dream property, become less afraid. People don't scare me as much as they used to. I need their approval less than ever before in my life.

It's been a year since my last drink. My life has become better, fuller, more fulfilling, and most of all: bigger.

Alcohol makes our life small. It makes us talk about all the things we want to do, but the more we drink the less likely we are to do them. Drinking is time-consuming, anxiety-producing, expensive and soul-destroying. It robs us of energy, creativity, courage, mindfulness, real connection, and peace.

I don't have the mindset that I don't *get* to drink anymore. On the contrary, I drink as much and as often as I want! Which happens to be zero, because I don't want it. I don't *have* to drink anymore.

These days I'm carrying around a secret that warms me instead of one that slowly destroys me. It makes me feel strong and empowered.

Remember my obsession with happiness I talked about at the beginning of this book?

I've found it. Happiness is freedom: the freedom to be who you truly are.

Acknowledgments

I would like to thank my two therapists Tori and Lola (not their real names). You have both completely transformed how I live with my mental illness.

The title of the book is a partial quote from the brilliant book *Sorrow and Bliss* by Meg Mason. I was listening to the audiobook during a walk and when I heard it (the full quote is *"Everything is broken and messed up and completely fine. That is what life is. It's only the ratios that change."*) it gave me a physical jolt of recognition. I knew right away that this is what I wanted to call my book.

I'm deeply grateful to the female authors who have inspired me with their work: Jeannette Walls whose bestselling memoir *The Glass Castle* is my favourite book of all time and made me fall in love with memoirs. Elizabeth Gilbert for *Big Magic*, the guiding light on my creative journey. Glennon Doyle for *Untamed*, a call to action for women to live life according to their own rules.

I will always be thankful to the sober community online and in literature for not only showing me the real face of alcohol but also how beautiful living an alcohol-free life is. I have gained knowledge, an expanded worldview and greater understanding for myself and others.

Lastly, all my love belongs to my husband Richard. When you said twenty years ago that you would always be there for me you sure meant it! We've gone through a lot together (no small thanks to my mental illness) but you never waver. Thank you for being by my side, always. I love you.

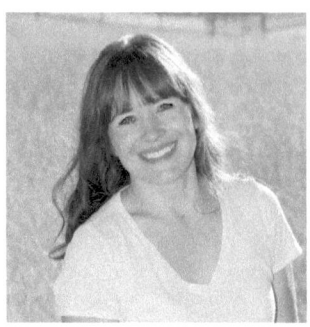

About the Author

Miriam Verheyden is a Canadian non-fiction writer, novelist, x-ray technologist, and mental health advocate.

Known for her honesty and deep vulnerability, she writes books about love, fear, mental health, sobriety, and being a woman in the world.

Miriam was born and raised in Germany. During a solo trip at 22 to the wild west of Canada she fell in love with her husband, dropped everything at home and moved to British Columbia to be with him. 20+ years later they are still happily married, living on a ranch in the interior of BC.

You can connect with me on:
- https://miriamverheyden.com
- https://www.facebook.com/miriamverheydenwriter
- https://www.instagram.com/miriamverheydenwriter

Subscribe to my newsletter:
- https://miriamverheyden.substack.com

Also by Miriam Verheyden

Miriam writes deeply vulnerable books about being a woman in the world.

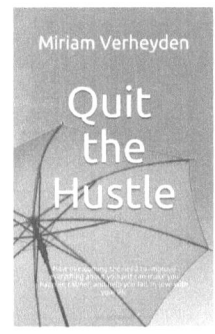

Quit the Hustle

Never has the hustle been more glorified than it is today. We have been told for decades that we have to do it all: have kids, a great relationship, a career, a Pinterest-worthy house and a perfect body and face. But with the rise of the #bossbabes even that is not enough anymore: we should also strive to turn our hobby into a side hustle, follow the latest healthy eating trends and pretend that celery juice tastes better than coffee. But the tide is turning. We are fed up with the chase for perfection. This book explores what happens when we stop doing and start being – and let me tell you, it's magical.

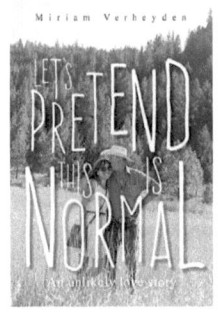

Let's Pretend This is Normal

Life after high school wasn't at all how Miriam imagined it. Instead of having big plans and excitement for the future, she had no idea what she wanted to do with her life and struggled to find her purpose. When the man she thought would save her from herself married her sister, she traveled to the Wild West of Canada on a journey of self-discovery and found much more than she bargained for: she fell head over heels in love with Richard, twenty-five years her senior and a father of four. When she introduced him to her shocked family, they tried to persuade her to leave him. Failing, they did the next best thing: they pretended it was normal.

Let's Pretend This Is Normal is a testament to what can happen when you listen to your heart instead of the opinions of others. This tale of romance and growing up is proof that even if you have no idea what the hell you're doing, with some patience and trust in yourself, you'll figure it out.

www.ingramcontent.com/pod-product-compliance
Lightning Source LLC
Chambersburg PA
CBHW060559080526
44585CB00013B/620